Fundamentals of Clinical Ophthalmology

Uveitis

Fundamentals of Clinical Ophthalmology

Uveitis

Susan Lightman
Department of Clinical Ophthalmology
Institute of Ophthalmology/Moorfields Eye Hospital,
London, UK

and

Hamish MA Towler
Consultant Ophthalmic Surgeon
Whipps Cross Hospital, London, UK

Series Editor:
Susan Lightman

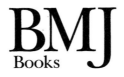

BMJ
Books

First published in 1998
by BMJ Books, BMA House, Tavistock Square
London WC1H 9JR

British Library Cataloguing in Publication Data

A catalogue record for this book is available from the British Library

ISBN 0-7279-1202-X

Typeset by Apek Typesetters, Nailsea, Bristol
Printed and bound by Craft Print Pte Ltd, Singapore

Contents

Acknowledgments

We would like to thank all of the ophthalmologists who have contributed to this book, many of whom have worked in the past as Fellows with the Uveitis Service at Moorfields Eye Hospital. We would also like to thank all the other people, too numerous to mention, who have also contributed in so many ways over the years.

Contributors

Keith Barton
Consultant Ophthalmologist
Moorfields Eye Hospital, London, UK

Diana Conrad
Consultant Ophthalmologist
Brisbane, Australia

Anthony J H Hall
Consultant Ophthalmologist
Melbourne, Australia

Susan Lightman
Professor of Clinical Ophthalmology
Moorfields Eye Hospital and Institute of Ophthalmology,
London, UK

P J McCluskey
Consultant Ophthalmologist
New South Wales, Australia

Carlos E Pavésio
Consultant Ophthalmologist
Moorfields Eye Hospital, London, UK

Hamish MA Towler
Consultant Ophthalmologist
Whipps Cross Hospital, London, UK

Preface to the *Fundamentals of Clinical Ophthalmology* series

This book is part of a series of ophthalmic monographs, written for ophthalmologists in training and general ophthalmologists wishing to update their knowledge in specialised areas. The emphasis of each is to combine clinical experience with the current knowledge of the underlying disease processes.

Each monograph provides an up to date, very clinical and practical approach to the subject so that the reader can readily use the information in everyday clinical practice. There are excellent illustrations throughout each text in order to make it easier to relate the subject matter to the patient.

The inspiration for the series came from the growth in communication and training opportunities for ophthalmologists all over the world and a desire to provide clinical books that we can all use. This aim is well reflected in the international panels of contributors who have so generously contributed their time and expertise.

Susan Lightman and Hamish Towler

Preface

The recognition of the different patterns of uveitis is dependent primarily upon basic clinical skills, relying on the acquisition of a careful ophthalmic and systematic history, supported by meticulous examination of the eye and other relevant systems. Investigations play a limited role in the corroboration of the distinct uveitis entities, but may be of great value when used selectively.

This book emphasises the clinical approach to uveitis, and aims to provide a practical guide to the diagnosis, differential diagnosis, and management of uveitis in all its manifestations. The illustrations have been carefully chosen to complement this clinical approach, and are supported by a balanced selection of references.

Susan Lightman and Hamish Towler

1: Anterior uveitis: differential diagnosis and management

Acute anterior uveitis is the most common form of intraocular inflammation and accounts for approximately three quarters of cases.[1] In a community setting, anterior uveitis may account for up to 90% of uveitis cases, whereas the proportion is lower in a tertiary referral centre.[2-4] The annual incidence is estimated to be between 8 and 20 new cases per 100 000 population.[5, 6] In up to 50% of cases no specific cause can be found[2] but, in all patients, associated systemic disease should be looked for.

Definitions

Inflammation confined primarily to the iris and anterior chamber is referred to as iritis. Cyclitis refers to inflammation affecting the ciliary body and anterior vitreous. Inflammation involving both the anterior chamber and anterior vitreous is termed "iridocyclitis". Anterior uveitis encompasses both iritis and iridocyclitis.

Anterior uveitis can be classified according to its time course. Acute anterior uveitis lasts days to weeks and resolves completely between episodes. Chronic uveitis lasts from months to years. The time course and anatomical localisation of uveitis help in the diagnosis and management of the patient.

CLINICAL FEATURES
Symptoms

Patients with acute anterior uveitis present with pain, typically a deep periorbital ache, redness, and photophobia. There may be

1

associated epiphora, especially in bright light. Patients with chronic anterior uveitis are usually less symptomatic.

Signs

The conjunctival injection associated with anterior uveitis is predominantly perilimbal, and is known as ciliary flush. The characteristic findings in acute anterior uveitis are cells and flare in the anterior chamber resulting from breakdown of the blood ocular barrier. Flare is caused by increased protein content in the aqueous, resulting in increased visibility of the slit beam (Tyndall effect). Cells are detected by observing the oblique slit beam and focusing between the corneal endothelium and the anterior iris or lens surface. The cell number is graded from 0 to 5 (Table 1.1). In severe cases, the cells appear static and suspended in the aqueous (plastic aqueous). Hypopyon occurs when the cells in the anterior chamber collect inferiorly, producing a white "level" (Fig 1.1). Flare is graded as 0–4, with grade 4 describing when fibrin deposition occurs within the anterior chamber.

Inflammatory cells deposited on the corneal endothelium are referred to as keratic precipitates (KPs). These have been segregated into granulomatous ("mutton fat") KPs, which are greasy looking, large KPs, which tend to cluster in the inferior one third of the cornea and may coalesce (Fig 1.2), and non-granulomatous KPs, which tend to be fine and small. The clinical distinction of granulomatous or non-granulomatous uveitis does not correlate well with histopathological findings[7] and is therefore not a useful concept. The KPs of Fuchs' heterochromic cyclitis are almost

Table 1.1 Grading of anterior chamber cells using 1 mm × 1 mm slit

Grade	Cells
0	0
Trace	1–5
1 +	6–15
2 +	16–25
3 +	26–50
4 +	>50

From Nussenblatt RB, Whitcup SM, Palestine AG. Examination of the patient with uveitis. In: *Uveitis Fundamentals and Clinical Practice*, 2nd edn. St Louis, MI: Mosby Year Book, 1996:56–68.

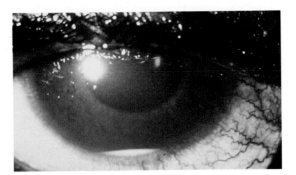

Figure 1.1   Hypoyon in acute uveitis.

pathognomonic, being small, non-pigmented, and dispersed evenly over the corneal endothelium. Nodules may occur on the iris and are divided into Koeppe nodules, which can be found around the pupil margin, and Busacca nodules, which occur in the iris stroma.

Adhesions may form between the iris and anterior lens surface (posterior synechiae) or the peripheral iris and the angle structures (peripheral anterior synechiae or PAS).

Intraocular pressure may be increased as a result of either angle closure secondary to pupil block or peripheral anterior synechiae, or inflammatory debris obstructing the trabecular outflow. Intraocular pressure may also be reduced as a result of severe inflammation affecting the ciliary body and reducing aqueous production or of ciliary body detachment caused by cyclitic membrane formation.

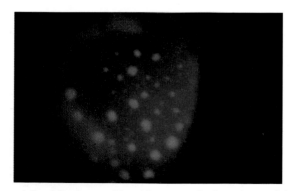

Figure 1.2   Anterior uveitis with mutton fat keratic precipitates.

3

History and physical examination

A complete general medical and ophthalmic history must be taken in the clinical setting of anterior uveitis. Specifically, previous rheumatic diseases, skin complaints, bowel problems, infections, use of medication, and sexual history should be investigated. A general examination should include examination of skin rashes or joint problems.

The ophthalmic history should concentrate on the current episode as well as any previous episodes of ocular inflammation, including their duration, response to therapy, and visual outcome. The pupils should be examined to detect any afferent defect, or pupil irregularity, and a thorough slitlamp examination performed. All patients with anterior uveitis should have a full dilated fundal examination with indirect ophthalmoscopy to determine whether there is any posterior segment involvement. Anterior segment inflammation can be quantified by using a laser flare cell meter.[8] This allows more standardised comparisons within and between patients and is especially useful in the research setting.[9-11]

DIFFERENTIAL DIAGNOSIS

Anterior uveitis can be divided into acute, chronic, and acute on chronic types; each has its own disease associations. Recognition of these different types can avoid unnecessary investigations and also inappropiate therapy.

Anterior uveitis associated with HLA-B27

The HLA-B27 antigen is a major histocompatibility complex class I molecule frequently associated with the seronegative spondyloarthropathies and uveitis.[12, 13] It is present in between 1.4% and 8.0% of the general population. Between 50% and 60% of patients with acute anterior uveitis are HLA-B27 positive. When the uveitis is unilateral and recurrent, as many as 71% of patients may be HLA-B27 positive.[14] Although anterior uveitis associated with HLA-B27 is a common cause of uveitis in the western world, it is less common in developing countries.[15] The precise trigger for acute anterior uveitis in genetically susceptible individuals is not clear.[16] Exposure to Gram negative organisms has been implicated in some patients.[17, 18] This group makes up the largest single group of patients with acute anterior uveitis. The diseases associated with HLA-B27 and anterior uveitis include: ankylosing spondylitis, inflammatory bowel disease (both Crohn's disease and ulcerative colitis), Reiter's syndrome, and psoriatic arthritis. Anterior uveitis can also occur in association with HLA-B27 positivity with no associated systemic disease.[19] In one study, 32% of patients had no associated systemic disease, and systemic disease may be undiagnosed before the onset of ocular disease.[20]

Ankylosing spondylitis

Ankylosing spondylitis affects 0.1% of white European adults, and is three times more common in men than in women. Ninety six per cent of patients are HLA-B27 positive, compared with 6% of the general population.[21]

Anterior uveitis affects 25% of patients with ankylosing spondylitis.[12] The inflammation is usually unilateral; however, in 80% both eyes will become involved at some time. The inflammation is acute, recurrent, and symptomatic, and usually responds rapidly to steroids. The arthropathy of ankylosing spondylitis varies from an asymptomatic condition to a severe, crippling disorder. Sacroiliitis is the most common systemic manifestation and presents as low back pain. Peripheral joints can also become involved in time, and these patients may be at greater risk for anterior uveitis.[22] Sacroiliac radiographs may show sclerosis of the joint space. Inflammation can involve the spine, which may result in eventual spinal fusion and the classic "bamboo spine" appearance on radiological examination. Rarely, ankylosing spondylitis may be associated with cardiac conduction disturbances, aortic insufficiency, and pulmonary apical fibrosis. It is important to make the systemic diagnosis of ankylosing spondylitis because early physiotherapy can help to maintain mobility.[23]

Ulcerative colitis

Ocular involvement, most commonly acute anterior uveitis, occurs in 5% of patients with ulcerative colitis. The ocular inflammation may assist in the diagnosis of the bowel disorder, so a gastroenterological history should be sought in these patients. Some patients with ulcerative colitis and anterior uveitis will also have radiological or clinical evidence of ankylosing spondylitis.

Crohn's disease

Five per cent of patients with Crohn's disease develop ocular complications, the most common of which is acute anterior uveitis. Other findings include episcleritis, scleritis, optic neuritis, extraocular muscle pareses, and lid oedema. Rarely, retinal vasculitis and peripheral corneal infiltrates may occur.

Reiter's syndrome

Rieter first described a triad of non-specific urethritis, conjunctivitis, and arthritis in 1916.[24] Conjunctivitis is the most frequent ocular finding and is usually transient. Twelve per cent of Reiter's syndrome patients develop mild non-granulomatous anterior uveitis, and less commonly keratitis with multifocal stromal and subepithelial punctate infiltrates. Pannus may develop. The anterior uveitis is usually responsive to steroids; it does tend to recur, however, and may rarely become chronic.

Reiter's syndrome may also be associated with keratoderma blenorrhagica—a scaling dermatitis of the hands and feet, aphthous stomatitis, balanitis, and arthritis. Eighty per cent of Reiter's syndrome patients are HLA-B27 positive. Reiter's syndrome may be precipitated by Gram negative dysentery caused by *Salmonella*, *Shigella*, or *Yersinia* species. It may also follow nongonococcal urethritis caused by *Chlamydia trachomatis* or *Ureaplasma urealyticum*.[25–27] Treatment of the urethritis does not appear to affect the course of the ocular disease.[28]

Psoriatic arthritis

Psoriasis is a chronic scaling dermatitis caused by hyperproliferation of the epidermis. A small proportion of people with psoriasis develop arthritis, which can involve the distal inter-phalangeal joints of the hands and feet. Acute anterior uveitis may occur in conjunction with psoriatic arthritis. Twenty per cent of patients with psoriatic arthritis may have sacroiliitis, and inflammatory bowel disease occurs more frequently than in control populations. Diagnosis is based on the typical cutaneous findings, distal interphalangeal joint inflammation, and nail changes. Treatment of the skin disease does not alter the course of the uveitis.

Anterior uveitis secondary to other rheumatic diseases

Sjögren's syndrome is an autoimmune disorder characterised by dry eye and dry mouth which has been associated with bilateral chronic anterior uveitis.[29] Anterior uveitis is an uncommon manifestation of rheumatoid arthritis, in which keratoconjunctivitis sicca, episcleritis, scleritis, and scleromalacia perforans are more characteristic. Patients with severe anterior scleritis may develop a secondary anterior uveitis.

Idiopathic anterior uveitis

Despite exhaustive history, examination, and laboratory investigation, many uveitis patients never receive a specific aetiological diagnosis. Even when followed for many years, these patients do not develop symptoms or signs of systemic inflammation. The most common diagnostic group is therefore this group of patients with idiopathic anterior uveitis. A prospective study of 865 uveitis patients found no associated systemic disease in 24%. A definite association with systemic disease was found in 23%. For 27% of patients no specific diagnosis could be determined.[30]

These patients present with pain, redness, and photophobia. The inflammation is associated with small KPs, significant anterior chamber cells and flare, and the development of posterior synechiae. The inflammation is usually unilateral, but may recur in the contralateral eye. It may be acute, recurrent, chronic, or acute on chronic.

Juvenile chronic arthritis

The most common cause of chronic anterior uveitis in children is juvenile chronic arthritis (JCA).[31] The risk for uveitis depends on the clinical presentation of the arthritis. The risk is greater in girls with the seronegative, antinuclear antibody (ANA) positive, pauciarticular form of JCA.[32] This group tends to develop a chronic bilateral anterior uveitis with a high incidence of band keratopathy, posterior synechiae, and cataract (Fig 1.3). The eye is usually white and non-inflamed in appearance, and there is little discomfort so its recognition may be delayed.

The prognosis is often poor, resulting partly from delay in diagnosis and treatment. Children with JCA should therefore be screened with regular slitlamp examinations to detect silent ocular damage. Chronic inflammation can result in peripheral anterior synechiae, posterior synechiae, glaucoma, cystoid macular oedema, and chronic calcific band keratopathy. Severe cases may develop cyclitic membranes, and may eventually go into phthisis.

Antibodies against ocular tissues have been identified in the serum of patients with JCA,[33] but their significance in the pathogenesis of ocular disease is unknown. Chronic iridocyclitis can also be seen, particularly in girls, without any association with JCA, and the course, prognosis, and treatment are very similar. In boys, it is necessary to distinguish the group with pauciarticular disease who are positive for HLA-B27. This group tends to develop acute, recurrent, ocular inflammation, as in adults with HLA-B27, and may go on to develop ankylosing spondylitis.[34]

Adult onset Still's disease may also be associated with persistent

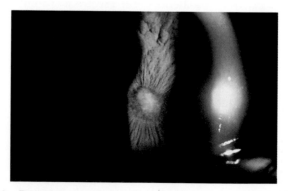

Figure 1.3   Bound down pupil with extensive posterior synechiae with cataract in a child with juvenile chronic arthritis.

chronic anterior uveitis. These patients present with fevers, polyarthritis and polymyalgia, and an evanescent macular rash.

Treatment

Treatment of JCA consists of topical steroids and, rarely, systemic or periocular steroids. Long term cycloplegia may be required to prevent posterior synechiae. Band keratopathy may require chelation therapy with ethylenediamine tetracetic acid (EDTA) or excimer laser phototherapeutic keratectomy (PTK) (see chapter 9).

Management of cataract in this patient group can be very difficult. Routine cataract surgery may be associated with a high incidence of complications. Consideration should be given to lensectomy—vitrectomy via a pars plana approach to prevent the formation of postoperative cyclitic membranes[35, 36] (see chapter 9).

Fuchs' heterochromic cyclitis

This disorder was first described by Fuchs in 1906.[37] This is a disease of unknown aetiology, characterised by chronic low grade anterior uveitis. Heterochromia is a prominent finding in this disorder. In patients with blue eyes, the involved eye appears a deeper blue.[38] In brown eyed patients the heterochromia may be very subtle. Atrophy of the anterior iris surface results in blunting of the iris rugae and an irregular pupil, and the pupil in the involved eye may be enlarged. There may be pigment epithelial atrophy of the iris resulting in transillumination defects. The anterior chamber usually has low grade cells and flare. The KPs in this disease are characteristic, and are fine, white, and stellate with fine filaments between the lesions, and widely distributed over the corneal endothelium (Fig 1.4). Anterior vitreous cells are also common. Koeppe nodules are occasionally seen, although posterior synechiae never form[39] unless the eye has undergone surgery. Abnormal vessels on the anterior iris surface and in the angle are seen in the chronic stages, and these tend to be friable. Amsler's sign has been described in these patients as a filiform haemorrhage in the chamber angle after paracentesis. This disease is usually unilateral, but may be bilateral in 10%, in whom heterochromia is difficult to detect.

Complications of this disease include cataract, characteristically

9

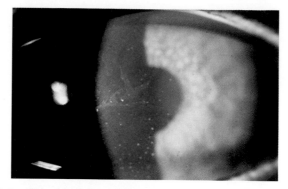

Figure 1.4 Characteristic appearance of iris nodules and keratic precipitates in Fuchs' heterochromic cyclitis.

a posterior subcapsular cataract, vitritis, and glaucoma, which occurs in about 25–33% of patients.[40] Patients are frequently asymptomatic, but may present with floaters at the time of posterior vitreous detachment, or decreased vision resulting from cataract.

The pathogenesis of this condition is unknown. It may be the end stage of a number of ocular insults, or a separate condition. Fuchs' heterochromic cyclitis has been associated with chorioretinal scars with the appearance of toxoplasmosis. Although originally thought to be associated,[41] further studies have shown that this is not the case.[42] Steroids do not affect the anterior uveitis or the course of the disease, and should not be used. Treatment is directed to that of the associated complications—cataract, vitritis, and glaucoma. These patients generally do well with routine cataract surgery, with intraocular lens implantation. They can develop anterior lens deposits, pigmented KPs and posterior synechiae postoperatively (Fig 1.5), and require topical steroids in the postoperative period. The prognosis is good in most cases, even though the inflammation may continue for decades.[43] Floaters may be a presenting problem or noticeable only after cataract extraction and may be helped significantly by vitrectomy. The glaucoma is usually managed with topical medication, but may occasionally be difficult to control, requiring further medication and/or surgery (see chapter 9).

The differential diagnosis of iris heterochromia should be considered in all patients with Fuchs' heterochromic cyclitis. Any chronic uveitis can result in a "moth-eaten" appearance to the iris, but the following should be particularly excluded: iris naevus, iris

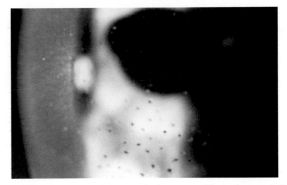

Figure 1.5   Posterior synechiae and pigmented keratic precipitates after Fuchs' heterochromic cyclitis after cataract surgery.

melanoma, melanosis bulbi, metallic siderosis, Horner's syndrome, and chronic iritis with secondary iris atrophy resulting from tuberculosis, syphilis, or herpes zoster.

Glaucomatocyclitic crisis (Posner–Schlossman syndrome)

Posner–Schlossman syndrome consists of intermittent recurrent attacks of low grade intraocular inflammation with associated elevated intraocular pressure. It is thought that the inflammation involves predominantly the trabecular meshwork. Fine KPs may be seen on the corneal endothelium and in the anterior chamber angle. The aetiology is not known, although recent evidence has suggested a possible role for herpes simplex virus in the origin of this condition.[44] Treatment is with topical steroids and cycloplegics, as well as β blockers and oral carbonic anhydrase inhibitors while the pressure is elevated. The episodes vary in their length from days to weeks.[45]

Sarcoidosis

Ocular complications occur in 20–50% of patients with sarcoidosis.[46] The most common manifestation is anterior uveitis. Anterior uveitis associated with sarcoidosis is characterised by

11

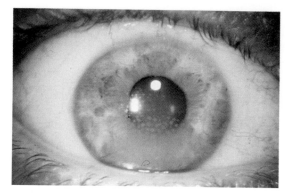

Figure 1.6 Anterior uveitis with large iris nodules and keratic precipitates as seen in sarcoidosis.

mutton fat KPs, iris nodules (Fig 1.6), extensive synechiae, and anterior chamber cells and flare. The inflammation is characteristically bilateral, but unilateral or asymmetrical inflammation can occur. The inflammation is most commonly chronic, but may be acute or recurrent. Ocular sarcoidosis may also involve the posterior segment, with vitritis, retinal periphlebitis, optic disc oedema, and cystoid macular oedema (see chapter 3).

Behçet's disease

Although Behçet's disease may involve the posterior segment, this inflammatory disorder may present initially as anterior uveitis. This is a chronic multisystem disorder that predominantly affects young males. Behçet was a Turkish dermatologist who described this syndrome in 1937.[47] The major triad of Behçet's disease is anterior uveitis, oral aphthous ulcers, and genital ulcers. Other features include arthropathy, thrombophlebitis, and erythema nodosum. Ocular manifestations occur in 70–85% of Behçet's disease patients.[48] The most common ocular manifestation is a severe anterior uveitis, often with hypopyon, which may be bilateral. There may be associated posterior segment involvement with obliterative retinal vasculitis (see chapter 6).

Multiple sclerosis

Chronic granulomatous anterior uveitis has been reported in association with multiple sclerosis. The more common form of ocular inflammation in this disease is intermediate uveitis (see chapter 3).[49]

Lens associated anterior uveitis

Phacoantigenic endophthalmitis is a dense granulomatous inflammation thought to represent an autoimmune response to lens proteins released into the anterior chamber. This disorder is seen after traumatic rupture of the lens capsule, either accidental or iatrogenic. The clinical features consist of lid oedema, conjunctival chemosis, and a severe anterior chamber reaction with mutton fat KPs, significant cells and flare, and anterior and posterior synechiae. Elevated intraocular pressure and cyclitic membranes may develop.

Treatment involves high dose topical, periocular, and systemic steroids, as well as therapy for any associated glaucoma. Infectious endophthalmitis should be considered in the differential diagnosis, especially in the setting of a penetrating eye injury.[50]

Phacolytic glaucoma is an anterior uveitis seen when a hypermature cataract has leaked liquefied cortex. It is characterised by a low grade anterior chamber reaction, with minimal KPs. The patient is only mildly symptomatic, unless the intraocular pressure becomes very elevated. Treatment involves frequent topical steroids and removal of the lens.[51]

Phacotoxic uveitis is thought to represent an overlap syndrome between phacoantigenic endophthalmitis and phacolytic glaucoma. Clinically, it is characterised by cells and flare in the anterior chamber with a variable number of keratic precipitates. Anterior and posterior synechiae may be present. The lens capsule may be intact or there may be a traumatic or surgical rupture. The inflammatory cells in the anterior segment include lymphocytes, monocytes, and neutrophils, with occasional giant cells.[52]

Pseudophakic iridocyclitis

In some patients, earlier types of lens implants were associated with a syndrome of uveitis, glaucoma, and hyphaema (UGH).

These anterior chamber lenses caused significant cell and flare, and occasional hypopyon and hyphaema. Glaucoma resulted from obstruction of the trabecular meshwork by inflammatory debris or red blood cells. This syndrome was particularly common with the early iris clip lenses. With present day lens implants, it is much less common. Intraocular lenses used to correct myopia in phakic eyes have been shown to cause a chronic increase in anterior chamber flare.[53]

Infectious causes of anterior uveitis

Infection must always be considered when a patient presents with uveitis of any type.

Viral

The virus most often implicated as a cause of anterior uveitis is herpes simplex virus type 1 (HSV1). Low grade anterior chamber inflammation may be seen as a complication of herpetic keratitis, especially with stromal involvement. Recurrent anterior chamber inflammation can be seen in the absence of keratitis. There may be associated severe elevations of intraocular pressure, presumably as a result of associated trabeculitis.

Herpetic keratouveitis should be treated with oral acyiclovir, and in some patients low dose maintenance treatment may be required to control frequent recurrences. Topical steroids are also usually required to control the intraocular inflammation with additional topical antivirals if there is active epithelial disease.

Ocular involvement is seen in two thirds of patients with herpes zoster involving the ophthalmic division of the trigeminal nerve.[54] The anterior chamber reaction develops some days after the initial appearance of the skin lesions, but it may precede, or occur in the absence of, the rash. It is postulated that this inflammation is caused by ciliary body ischaemia, as well as an inflammatory response to varicella antigen. Zoster associated uveitis may become chronic, and can be complicated by secondary glaucoma.

A low grade anterior uveitis may be seen in patients with cytomegalovirus (CMV) retinitis. Fine KPs and low grade cells and flare may be seen. If there is significant inflammation the diagnosis should be reviewed, although new drug therapies (for example, systemic protease inhibitors or cidofovir) may be associated with increased ocular inflammation.

Epstein–Barr virus (EBV) may be associated with anterior uveitis. This can occur at the time of the initial illness, or as a recurrent inflammation years later. Conjunctivitis and keratitis are also complications of this infection.

Bacterial

Chlamydial infection affects the conjunctiva and cornea primarily, with secondary anterior chamber inflammation appearing in some patients.

Delayed onset postoperative endophthalmitis after extracapsular cataract extraction with posterior chamber intraocular lens implantation has been reported in a number of cases to be caused by *Propionibacterium acnes*[55]—a Gram positive, anaerobic, pleomorphic rod. This infection may resemble postoperative anterior uveitis. It may occur as early as 2 weeks after surgery, and as late as 1 year. The characteristic finding is the development of capsular plaques (Fig 1.7). There may be transient improvement with topical steroids and the diagnosis requires a high index of suspicion. Therapy involves diagnostic aqueous and vitreous aspirates to identify the organism, and intravitreal antibiotics. Total capsulectomy and removal of the intraocular lens may be required to eradicate the infection because sequestration of the infection often occurs within the capsule (Fig 1.8).

Endogenous endophthalmitis presenting as anterior uveitis has been reported with *Listeria monocytogenes*, *Neisseria meningitidis*, and *Haemophilus influenzae*.

Mycoplasma pneumoniae is an atypical bacterium that is associated with respiratory infection, and may occasionally be

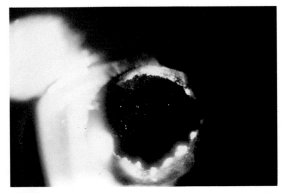

Figure 1.7 White plaques on the capsule in chronic endophthalmitis caused by *P. acnes*.

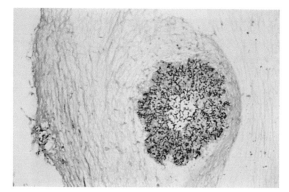

Figure 1.8   Silver stain to show *P. acnes* bacilli on capsulectomy specimen.

associated with a mild anterior uveitis.[56] The uveitis responds with treatment of the underlying infection.

The secondary stage of syphilis infection may be associated with a florid anterior uveitis with KPs which is usually bilateral. This inflammation may not respond to steroids. Syphilis should be considered in the differential diagnosis of any patient with progressive intraocular inflammation despite steroid therapy.

Mycobacterium leprae and *Mycobacterium tuberculosis* may both be associated with anterior uveitis. Systemic leprosy has a very high incidence of ocular complications,[57] and 5% of affected patients will eventually be blinded by the disease. The uveitis occurs in two forms: a chronic anterior uveitis associated with diffuse or segmental iris atrophy and progressive miosis, and an acute recurrent anterior uveitis.

Ocular tuberculosis may be associated with acute or chronic anterior uveitis, and there may be posterior segment involvement with retinal periphlebitis, vitritis, and occasionally, in disseminated infection, choroidal tubercles.[58]

Parasitic

Both toxoplasmosis and toxocariasis may be associated with a severe anterior segment inflammation (see chapter 5).

AIDS and anterior uveitis

A number of infections may affect the anterior segment in acquired immune deficiency syndrome (AIDS).[59] Cytomegalovirus infection may be associated with a low grade iridocyclitis. Reactivation of toxoplasmosis may cause a profound anterior chamber reaction in AIDS. *Toxoplasma gondii* cysts have been documented histopathologically within the iris in immunocompromised patients with anterior uveitis,[60] suggesting that the anterior uveitis in immunocompromised patients may involve direct infection of the iris and ciliary body by the parasite, rather than a secondary hypersensitivity reaction to posterior segment activation.

Syphilis may present with anterior segment inflammation in AIDS.[61] This may progress to retinal vasculitis, vitritis, optic neuritis, subretinal infiltrates, or acute retinitis.

Anterior uveitis in AIDS may be a direct manifestation of human immunodeficiency virus (HIV) infection, or an autoimmune process resulting from immune dysfunction. Reiter's syndrome may produce conjunctivitis and anterior uveitis in AIDS patients.[62] Drugs used in patients with complications of AIDS may also cause anterior uveitis (see below).

HTLV-1 associated uveitis

Human T lymphotrophic virus type 1 (HTLV-1) is a human retrovirus that is highly endemic in some regions of the world, and known to be a causative agent of T cell malignancies, progressive myelopathy, and uveitis. The most common ocular manifestation is a bilateral intermediate uveitis; however, patients may have an associated anterior uveitis, or peripheral retinal vasculitis.[63, 64]

Rare systemic associations

These are legion and too numerous to list. However, some in particular give an anterior uveitis rather than a panuveitis, for example, Kawasaki's disease,[65] in which two thirds of patients had evidence of anterior uveitis.[66] Interstitial nephritis, an uncommon form of renal disease that may occur after therapy with antibiotics or non-steroidal anti-inflammatory drugs (NSAIDs), may be associated with bilateral anterior uveitis particularly in women and children. The ocular involvement may precede or follow the renal disease.[67, 68]

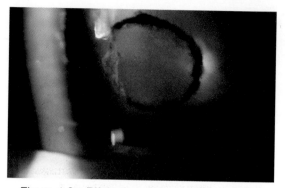

Figure 1.9   Rifabutin induced anterior uveitis.

Drugs and anterior uveitis

Rifabutin, a drug used to treat *Mycobacterium avium intracellulare* complex (MAC) infections in patients with AIDS has been found to be associated with the development of anterior uveitis (Fig 1.9). In higher doses it can cause panophthalmitis, with hypopyon. The inflammation is usually bilateral and responds rapidly to steroids and discontinuation of the medication.[69–71] More recently this has also been shown to be a complication of cidofovir treatment for CMV retinitis, when given intravenously or intravitreally.[72, 73]

Some topical glaucoma medications have also been associated with the development of anterior uveitis. Metipranolol has been associated with the development of granulomatous anterior uveitis.[74]

Pamidronate, an inhibitor of bone resorption that is used primarily in the management of tumour induced hypercalcaemia and Paget's disease, has been associated with the development of anterior uveitis.[75]

Case reports have implicated other drugs, such as sulphonamides, as causes of acute anterior uveitis.[76, 77]

Anterior segment ischaemia

Anterior segment ischaemia caused by severe carotid insufficiency may simulate an anterior uveitis in older patients. Patients develop an anterior uveitis with flare out of proportion to the cellular response. The pupil may be sluggish, and there is often significant pain. There may be other signs of ischaemia, including venous stasis and neovascularisation.[78]

Masquerade syndromes

Masquerade syndromes are diseases that may present as uveitis but have an underlying cause such as infection (see above) or malignancy.[79] Anterior uveitis that is unresponsive to steroids in an elderly person may result from intraocular lymphoma (Fig 1.10). Diagnosis is made by cytological examination of aqueous or vitreous humour.[80] Most cases of intraocular lymphoma present with bilateral uveitis that is predominantly posterior (see chapter 2).

Acute relapses of leukaemia may present with anterior segment leukaemic infiltrate which may be difficult to distinguish from acute anterior uveitis.[81, 82] Retinoblastoma may present with a pseudohyopyon caused by a collection of malignant cells in the anterior chamber.

MANAGEMENT

Classically, an attack of anterior uveitis will last from several days to 6 weeks. The attacks are usually unilateral, but may alternate

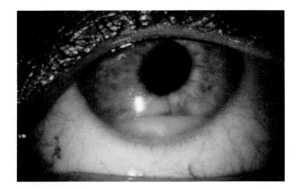

Figure 1.10   Hyoypon in lymphoma masquerading as a uveitis.

between the two eyes. Recurrences are common, but rarely bilateral. Corticosteroids are the mainstay of treatment for anterior uveitis. These reduce inflammation, prevent scarring, and minimise damage to the uveal vasculature. Topical drops are used initially, with a frequency up to every hour during the day, with steroid ointment supplementation at night. Occasionally, periocular steroid injections are required and, in severe cases, oral steroids. Very rarely, if ever is immunosuppressive therapy required. Early reports suggest that topical non-steroidal anti-inflammatory drugs may have a role to play in the management of mild anterior uveitis, but steroids remain the treatment of choice.[83, 84] Patients on chronic therapy should be maintained on the weakest topical steroid preparation that can reasonably control the inflammation and steroid responders (patients in whom the 108 mixes when topical steriods are administrated) should be watched for.

Cycloplegia is used to relieve pain from iris spasm, and to break down and prevent synechiae formation. Cycloplegics may be administered as topical drops, in cotton soaked pledgets in the conjunctiva, or as subconjunctival injections. Initially longer acting cycloplegics, such as atropine and cyclopentolate, are used but these can be reduced to much shorter acting drugs, such as tropicamide, which can be used at night to prevent problems with accommodation occuring during the day.

1 Wakefield D, Dunlop I, McCluskey PJ. Uveitis: Aetiology and disease associations in an Australian population. *Aust NZ J Ophthalmol* 1986;14:181–7.

2 McCannel CA, Holland GN, Helm CJ, Cornell PJ, Winston JV, Rimmer TG. Causes of uveitis in the general practice of ophthalmology. UCLA Community-Based Uveitis Study Group. *Am J Ophthalmol* 1996;121:35–46.

3 Pivetti-Pezzi P, Accorinti M, La Cava M, Colabelli Gisoldi RA, Abdulaziz MA. Endogenous uveitis: an analysis of 1,417 cases. *Ophthalmologica* 1996;210:234–8.

4 Rodriguez A, Calonge M, Pedroza-Seres M, et al. Referral patterns of uveitis in a tertiary eye care center. *Arch Ophthalmol* 1996;114:593–9.

5 Rothova A, van Veendaal WG, Linssen A. Clinical features of acute anterior uveitis. *Am J Ophthalmol* 1987;103:137–45.

6 Saari KM, Paivonsalo-Hietanen T, Vaahtoranta-Lehtonen H, Tuominen J, Sillanpaa M. Epidemiology of endogenous uveitis in south-western Finland. *Acta Ophthalmol Scand* 1995;73:345–9.

7 Smith RE, Nozik NE. *Uveitis: Fundamentals and clinical practices.* Baltimore, MA: Williams & WIlkins, 1989.

8 Sawa M. Clinical application of laser flare-cell meter. *Jpn J Ophthalmol* 1990;34:346–63.

9 de Ancos E, Pittet N, Herbort CP. Quantitative measurement of inflammation in HLA-B27 acute anterior uveitis using the Kowa FC-100 laser flare-cell meter. *Klin Monats Augenheilk* 1994;204:330–3.

10 Guex-Crosier Y, Pittet N, Herbort CP. Evaluation of laser flare-cell photometry

in the appraisal and management of intraocular inflammation in uveitis. *Ophthalmology* 1994;**101**:728–35.

11 Herbort CP, Guex-Crosier Y, de Ancos E, Pittet N. Use of laser flare photometry to assess and monitor inflammation in uveitis. *Ophthalmology* 1997;**104**:64–71.

12 Brewerton DA, Caffrey M, Hart FD. Ankylosing spondylitis and HLA-27. *Lancet* 1973;**i**:904–7.

13 Kellner H, Yu D. The pathogenetic aspects of spondyloarthropathies from the point of view of HLA-B27. *Rheumatol Int* 1992;**12**:121–7.

14 Rosenbaum JT. Characterization of uveitis associated with spondylarthropathies. *J Rheumatol* 1989;**16**:792–6.

15 Ronday MJ, Stilma JS, Barbe RF, et al. Aetiology of uveitis in Sierra Leone, west Africa. *Br J Ophthalmol* 1996;**80**:956–61.

16 Wakefield D, Montanaro A, McCluskey P. Acute anterior uveitis and HLA-B27. *Surv Ophthalmol* 1991;**36**:223–32.

17 White L, McCoy R, Tait B, Ebringer R. A search for gram-negative enteric micro-organisms in acute anterior uveitis: Association of klebsiella with recent onset of disease, HLA-B27, and B7 CREG. *Br J Ophthalmol* 1984;**68**:750–5.

18 Sprenkels SH, Uksila J, Vainionpaa R, Toivanen P, Feltkamp TE. IgA antibodies in HLA-B27 associated acute anterior uveitis and ankylosing spondylitis. *Clin Rheumatol* 1996;**15**(Suppl 1):52–6.

19 Careless D, Inman RD. Acute anterior uveitis: clinical and experimental aspects. *Semin Arthr Rheum* 1995;**24**:432–41.

20 Tay-Kearney ML, Schwam BL, Lowder C, Ebringer R, Meisler DM, Vitale S. Clinical features and associated systemic diseases of HLA-B27 uveitis. *Am J Ophthalmol* 1996;**121**:47–56.

21 Masi AT. Epidemiology of B27 associated disease. *Ann Rheum Dis* 1979;**38**:131–4.

22 Maksymowych WP, Chou CT, Russell AS. Matching prevalence of peripheral arthritis and acute anterior uveitis in individuals with ankylosing spondylitis. *Ann Rheum Dis* 1995;**54**:128–30.

23 Calabro JJ, Eyvazzadeh C, Weber CA. Contemporary management of ankylosing spondylitis. *Compr Ther* 1986;**12**:11–18.

24 Reiter H. Über eine bisher unerkannte Spirochäteninsektion. *Dtsche Med Wochenschr* 1916;**42**:1535–6.

25 Dawson CR, Schachter J, Ostler HB. Inclusion conjunctivitis in Reiter's syndrome in a married couple. *Arch Ophthalmol* 1970;**83**:300.

26 Dawson CR, Schachter J. TRIC agent infections of the eye and genitatract. *Am J Ophthalmol* 1967;**63**:1288.

27 Catterall RD. Uveitis, arthritis, and non-specific genital infection. *Br J Vener Dis* 1960;**37**:27.

28 Keat A. Reiter's syndrome and reactive arthritis in perspective. *N Engl J Med* 1983;**39**:1606–15.

29 Rosenbaum JT, Bennett RM. Chronic anterior and posterior uveitis and primary Sjögren's syndrome. *Am J Ophthalmol* 1987;**104**:346–52.

30 Rothova A, Buitenhuis HJ, Meenken C, Brinkman CJ, Linssen A, Alberts C. Uveitis and systemic disease. *Br J Ophthalmol* 1992;**76**:137–41.

31 Pivetti-Pezzi P. Uveitis in children. *Eur J Ophthalmol* 1996;**6**:293–8.

32 Cassidy JT, Levinson JE, Bass JC. A study of classification criteria for a diagnosis of juvenile rheumatoid arthritis. *Arthritis Rheum* 1986;**29**:274–81.

33 Bloom JN, Ni M, Moore TL, Osborn TG, Hageman GS. Serum antiocular antibodies in patients with juvenile rheumatoid arthritis. *J Pediatr Ophthalmol Strabis* 1993;**30**:243–8.

34 Smiley WK. The eye in juvenile rheumatoid arthritis. *Trans Ophthalmol Soc UK* 1974;**94**:817–29.

35 Flynn HW, Davis JL, Culbertson WW. Pars plana lensectomy and vitrectomy for

complicated cataracts in juvenile rheumatoid arthritis. *Ophthalmology* 1988;**95**:1114–19.

36 Kanski JJ. Juvenile arthritis and uveitis. *Surv Ophthalmol* 1990;**95**:1247–51.

37 Fuchs E. Uber Komplikationen der Heterochromie. *Z Augenheilk* 1906;**15**:191–212.

38 Kimura SJ, Hogan MJ, Thygeson P. Fuchs' syndrome of heterochromic cyclitis. *Arch Ophthalmol* 1955;**54**:179–86.

39 Rothova A, La Hey E, Baarsma GS, Breebaart AC. Iris nodules in Fuchs' heterochromic uveitis. *Am J Ophthalmol* 1994;**118**:338–42.

40 Jones NP. Glaucoma in Fuchs' Heterochromic Uveitis: aetiology, management and outcome. *Eye* 1991;**5**:662–7.

41 De Abreu MT, Belfort R, Hirata PS. Fuchs' heterochromic iridocyclitis and ocular toxoplasmosis. *Am J Ophthalmol* 1982;**93**:739–44.

42 La Hey E, Rothova A, Baarsma GS, de Vries J, van Knapen F, Kijlstra A. Fuchs' heterochromic iridocyclitis is not associated with ocular toxoplasmosis. *Arch Ophthalmol* 1992;**110**:806–11.

43 Jones NP. Fuchs' heterochromic uveitis: a reappraisal of the clinical spectrum. *Eye* 1991;**5**:649–61.

44 Yamamoto S, Pavan-Langston D, Tada R, Yamamoto R, Kinoshita S, Nishida K. Possible role of herpes simplex virus in the origin of Posner–Schlossman syndrome. *Am J Ophthalmol* 1995;**119**:796–8.

45 Posner A, Schlossman A. Syndrome of unilateral recurrent attacks of glaucoma with cyclitis syndromes. *Arch Ophthalmol* 1948;**39**:517–28.

46 Obenoff CB, Shaw HE, Sydnor CF. Sarcoidosis and its ophthalmic manifestations. *Am J Ophthalmol* 1978;**86**:648–55.

47 Behçet H. Uber rez idivierende, aphthose durch ein virus verusachte Geschwure am Munde, am Auge und am Genitalen. *Dermatol Wochenschr* 1937;**105**:1152–7.

48 Michelson JB, Chisiari FV. Behçet's disease. *Surv Ophthalmol* 1984;**26**:190–203.

49 Acar MA, Birch MK, Abbott R, Rosenthal AR. Chronic granulomatous anterior uveitis associated with multiple sclerosis. *Graefes Arch Clin Exp Ophthalmol* 1993;**231**:166–8.

50 Apple DJ, Mamalis M, Steinmetz RL. Phacoanaphylactic endophthalmitis associated with extracapsular cataract extraction and posterior chamber intraocular lens. *Arch Ophthalmol* 1984;**102**:1528–32.

51 Verstad SL, Price PK, Hasland KR, Kaiser RB. Phacolytic glaucoma after extracapsular cataract extraction. *Glaucoma* 1983;**5**:206–9.

52 Irvine SR, Irvine ARJ. Lens-induced uveitis and glaucoma, part II: The phacotoxic reaction. *Am J Ophthalmol* 1952;**35**:370.

53 Perez–Santonja JJ, Iradier MT, Benitez del Castillo JM, Serrano JM, Zato MA. Chronic subclinical inflammation in phakic eyes with intraocular lenses to correct myopia. *J Cataract Refract Surg* 1996;**22**:183–7.

54 Womack LW, Liesegang TJ. Complications of herpes zoster ophthalmicus. *Arch Ophthalmol* 1983;**101**:42–5.

55 Winward KE, Pflugfelder SC, Flynn HW, Roussel TJ, Davis JL. Post-operative Propionibacterium endophthalmitis: treatment strategies and long-term results. *Ophthalmol* 1993;**100**:447–51

56 Dawidek GM. Anterior uveitis associated with *Mycoplasma pneumoniae* pneumonia. *Postgrad Med J* 1991;**67**:380–2.

57 Ffytche TGA. Iritis in leprosy. *Trans Ophthalmol Soc UK* 1981;**101**:325–7.

58 Garrow RW. Acute tuberculous pan-ophthalmitis. *Arch Ophthalmol* 1967;**78**:51–4.

59 Shuler JD, Engstrom RE, Holland GN. External ocular disease and anterior segment disorders associated with AIDS. *Int Ophthalmol Clin* 1989;**29**:98–104.

60 Rehder JR, Burnier M, Pavesio CE. Acute unilateral toxoplasmic iridocycliis in

AIDS patients. *Am J Ophthalmol* 1988;**106**:740–1.
61 Passo MS, Rosenbaum JT. Ocular syphilis is patients with human immunodeficiency virus infection. *Am J Ophthalmol* 1988;**106**:1–6.
62 Winchester R, Bernstein DH, Fischer HD. The co-occurrence of Reiter's syndrome in acquired immunodeficiency. *Ann Intern Med* 1987;**106**:19–26.
63 Yoshimura K, Mochizuki M, Araki S, et al. Clinical and immunological features of human T-cell lymphotropic virus type 1 uveitis. *Am J Ophthalmol* 1993;**116**:156–63.
64 Merle H, Smadja D, Le Hoang P, et al. Ocular manifestations in patients with HTLV-I associated infection—a clinical study of 93 cases. *Jpn J Ophthalmol* 1996;**40**:260–70.
65 Kawasaki T, Kosaki S, Okawa S. A new infantile mucocutaneous lymph node syndrome (MLNS) prevailing in Japan. *Pediatrics* 1974;**54**:271.
66 Burns JC, Joffe L, Sargent RA. Anterior uveitis associated with Kawasaki syndrome. *Pediatr Infect Dis* 1985;**4**:258–61.
67 Rodriguez-Perez JC, Cruz-Alamo M, Perez-Aciego P, Macia-Heras M, Naranjo-Hernandez A. Clinical and immune aspects of idiopathic acute tubulointerstitial nephritis and uveitis syndrome. *Am J Nephrol* 1995;**15**:386–91.
68 Smith RE, Alves-Filho G, Ribeiro-Alves MA. Acute tubulointerstitial nephritis and uveitis with antineutrophil cytoplasmic antibody. *Am J Kidney Dis* 1996;**28**:124–7.
69 Jacobs DS, Piliero PJ, Kuperwaser MG. Acute uveitis associated wiht rifabutin use in patients with human immunodeficiency virus infection. *Am J Ophthalmol* 1994;**118**:716–22.
70 Saran BR, Maguire AM, Nichols C. Hypopyon uveitis in patients with acquired immunodeficiency syndrome treated for systemic Mycobacterium avium complex infection with rifabutin. *Am J Ophthalmol* 1994;**112**:1159–65.
71 Schimkat M, Althaus C, Becker K, Sundmacher R. Rifabutin-associated anterior uveitis in patients with human immunodeficiency virus. *German J Ophthalmol* 1996;**5**:195–201.
72 Davis JL, Taskintuna I, Freeman WR, Weinberg DV, Feuer WJ, Leonard RE Iritis and hypotony after treatment with intravenous cidofovir for cytomegalovirus retinitis *Arch Ophthalmol* 1997;**115**:733–7.
73 Taskintuna I, Rahhal FM, Arevalo JF, Munguia D, Banker AS, De Clercq E, Freeman WR. Low-dose intravitreal cidofovir (HPMPC) therapy of cytomegalovirus retinitis in patients with acquired immune deficiency syndrome. *Ophthalmology* 1997; **104**:1049–57.
74 Burvenich H. Metipranolol associated granulomatous anterior uveitis: not so uncommon as thought. *Bull Soc Belge d'Ophtalmol* 1995;**257**:63–6.
75 Macarol V, Fraunfelder FT. Pamidronate disodium and possible ocular adverse drug reactions. *Am J Ophthalmol* 1994;**118**:220–4.
76 Northrop CV, Shepherd SM, Abbuhl S. Sulfonamide-induced iritis. *Am J Emerg Med* 1996;**14**:577–9.
77 Tilden ME, Rosenbaum JT, Fraunfelder FT. Systemic sulfonamides as a cause of bilateral, anterior uveitis. *Arch Ophthalmol* 1991;**109**:67–9.
78 Jacobs NA, Ridgway AE. Syndrome of ischaemic ocular inflammation: Six cases and a review. *Br J Ophthalmol* 1985;**69**:682–7.
79 Zamiri P, Boyd S, Lightman S. Uveitis in the elderly—is it easy to identify the masquerade? *Br J Ophthalmol* 1997, in press.
80 Char DH, Ljung B-M, Miller T, Phillips T. Primary intraocular lymphoma: diagnosis and management. *Ophthalmology* 1988;**95**:625–30.
81 Badeeb O, Anwar M, Farwan K, Tashkandi I, Omar A, Marzouki A. Leukemic infiltrate versus anterior uveitis. *Ann Ophthalmol* 1992;**24**:295–8.
82 Ayliffe W, Foster CS, Marcoux P, et al. Relapsing acute myeloid leukemia manifesting as hypopyon uveitis. *Am J Ophthalmology* 1995;**119**:361–4.

83 Foster CS, Alter G, DeBarge LR, et al. Efficacy and safety of rimexolone 1% ophthalmic suspension vs 1% prednisolone acetate in the treatment of uveitis. *Am J Ophthalmol* 1996;**122**:171–82.

84 Dunne JA, Jacobs N, Morrison A, Gilbert DJ. Efficacy in anterior uveitis of two known steroids and topical tolmetin. *Br J Ophthalmol* 1985;**69**:120–5

2: Intermediate uveitis

The term "intermediate uveitis" was introduced by the International Uveitis Study Group as part of its anatomical classification of uveitis[1] and defines inflammation centred on the pars plana, choroid, and peripheral retina. Pars planitis is a type of intermediate uveitis in which there is a characteristic accumulation of inflammatory material in the region of the vitreous base and pars plana; this is termed a "snowbank". Intermediate uveitis and pars planitis can be considered as similar diseases because they each define a similar clinical process. Patients with pars planitis may develop complications specifically related to the snowbank. The term "intermediate uveitis" has replaced terms such as posterior cyclitis, chronic cyclitis, and peripheral uveitis.

Intermediate uveitis is one of the most common uveitic syndromes involving the posterior segment, and accounts for up to 20% of patients with uveitis in series reported in the literature.[2] It occurs far more frequently than its published incidence would suggest, because there are a significant number of patients with mild disease who do not seek medical attention. Intermediate uveitis has a worldwide distribution and can occur at any age. There is no known racial or genetic predisposition. Familial occurrence is rare but recognised without a definite inheritance pattern.[3] Males and females are equally affected. Intermediate uveitis begins most commonly in children and young adults; it may be idiopathic in origin or occur in association with a number of systemic diseases and its diagnosis rests on its clinical signs.

Intermediate uveitis is a bilateral disease in more than 80% of patients, but up to 33% of patients present with unilateral disease. Many patients who present with uniocular symptoms have signs of intermediate uveitis in the other eye and most develop bilateral symptamatic disease with time. Uveitis involving the intermediate zone and pars plana can occur as an idiopathic process or as a manifestation of systemic diseases such as multiple sclerosis, sarcoidosis, tuberculosis, syphilis, Lyme disease, HIV infection, HTLV-1 infection, and inflammatory bowel disease. Ocular lymphoma may present with clinical signs similar to those of intermediate uveitis.

Intermediate uveitis may persist for many years before resolving and the great majority of patients have an excellent visual outcome. In a small number of patients severe ocular complications and visual loss can develop as a result of severe chronic inflammation.

PATHOLOGY AND PATHOGENESIS

Histopathological information on intermediate uveitis is limited and has come from eyes enucleated for complications of advanced disease and from surgical vitrectomy specimens. The vitreous of eyes enucleated with severe intermediate uveitis is infiltrated with mononuclear inflammatory cells.[4] Snowbanks are composed of fibroglial material (Fig 2.1) which has been laid down over the pars plana and vitreous base; this is adherent to the retina and may become vascularised by the retinal vessels.[5] There is an infiltrate of lymphocytes and fibrous astrocytes. Snowbanks probably represent reactive gliosis produced by Müller's cells (retinal glial cells). In the retina there may be optic disc swelling, macular oedema, and perivascular mononuclear cell cuffing of retinal blood vessels. There is a low grade inflammation in the ciliary body and a patchy peripheral choroiditis. The retinal inflammatory changes are often more marked than those seen in the uveal tract.

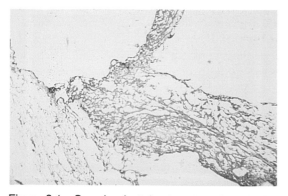

Figure 2.1   Snowbank stained to show glial tissue.

Immunohistochemistry of eyes enucleated with intermediate uveitis has revealed that the cellular infiltrate in intermediate uveitis consists predominantly of activated T cells, and most of these cells are CD4 + T cells.[5] CD8 + T cells, B cells, and macrophages are also present. There is increased expression of class II HLA antigens.

Vitrectomy specimens from eyes with intermediate uveitis have revealed a mixed infiltrate of T cells, B cells, macrophages, and giant cells.[4] Vitreous snowballs contain macrophages, epithelioid cells, and giant cells. Different populations of cells have been seen in different studies and are related to the stage of the disease at which the vitrectomy was performed.

The few available histological studies reveal that intermediate uveitis is characterised by a chronic inflammatory response consisting of T cells, macrophages, giant cells, and epithelioid cells. Retinal perivasculitis is also a prominent feature. The cause of the inflammation is unknown.

Recently, a 36 kDa protein (p-36 or nup 36) has been identified in the plasma of patients with pars planitis.[6] Its concentration is highest in patients with active disease. The protein p-36 has not been found in patients with other eye diseases, but has been found in patients with primary biliary cirrhosis and leukaemia. At this time the role of p-36 in the pathogenesis of pars planitis is unknown. The deduced amino acid sequence of the protein shows high sequence homology with the carboxy terminal region of a yeast nucleopore protein (nup 100). The significance of this is uncertain at this time, but available data suggest that p-36 is a human derived protein and may be part of a larger protein complex.[7, 8]

There are no clearly defined immunogenic markers for intermediate uveitis. One study has documented a 68% incidence of HLA-DR2 in patients with intermediate uveitis, compared with a 28% incidence in the control population.[9] This is of uncertain clinical significance at this time.

CLINICAL FEATURES

The onset of symptoms in patients with intermediate uveitis is usually vague and poorly characterised by the patient. Patients may complain of floaters, blurred vision, or reduced vision. Symptoms

27

may be unilateral or bilateral and often fluctuate. Intermediate uveitis is commonly asymptomatic and diagnosed at a routine eye examination, or if the patient develops complications such as symptomatic posterior vitreous detachment or vitreous haemorrhage. Patients may also present acutely with symptoms of anterior uveitis such as pain and photophobia.

The external eye is white and non-inflamed in most patients with intermediate uveitis. The anterior segment is quiet or has low grade flare and cells with a few keratic precipitates (KPs). Some patients present acutely with marked anterior uveitis. Posterior synechiae are uncommon, and the intraocular pressure is usually normal. Cataract may be present. A rare form of acute corneal endotheliitis may occur.[10]

The major signs of intermediate uveitis develop within the vitreous humour where there is a prominent cellular infiltrate and aggregations of cells inferiorly termed "vitreous snowballs" (Fig 2.2). The cellular infiltrate is usually most dense in the posterior vitreous. There are degenerative changes in the vitreous humour, such as synkinesis syneresis and posterior vitreous detachment. In severe pars planitis, inflammation may induce significant fibrocellular proliferation and traction within the vitreous humour and snowbanks.

The other major findings involve the retina and include: cystoid

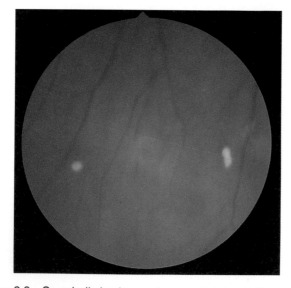

Figure 2.2   Snowballs in vitreous humour in intermediate uveitis.

macular oedema, optic disc swelling, diffuse retinal oedema, retinal vascular sheathing, and neovascularisation. Macular oedema is a prominent feature of intermediate uveitis and is the most common cause of visual loss. Chronic cystoid macular oedema may become irreversible as a result of permanent destruction of photoreceptors, retinal pigment epithelium destruction, or macular cyst/hole formation. There may be epiretinal membrane formation in association with macular oedema (Fig 2.3). In selected patients fluorescein angiography is useful in determining whether macular pathology is present and in evaluating its severity. Optic disc oedema is common in patients with active intermediate uveitis but seldom results in visual loss. Diffuse retinal oedema is common; widespread capillary closure and retinal ischaemic changes are not features of intermediate uveitis. There may be areas of venous sheathing in the peripheral retina and retinal neovascularisation involving the peripheral retina or optic disc (Fig 2.4). Retinal neovascularisation most commonly develops in the absence of retinal non-perfusion and is thought to be secondary to angiogenic inflammatory mediators. The choroid is normal and uninvolved in patients with intermediate uveitis. Patients with intermediate uveitis may have additional signs related to the development of complications such as cataract, glaucoma, vitreous haemorrhage, and retinal detachment.

In patients with pars planitis, in addition to the signs of

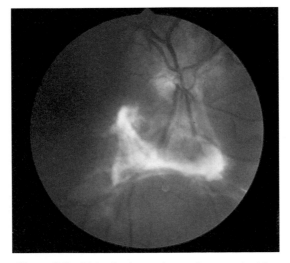

Figure 2.3   Epiretinal membrane in pars planitis.

29

intermediate uveitis, there are characteristic snowbanks which overlie the pars plana and adjacent peripheral retina. Snowbanks are elevated, white in colour (see Fig 2.4 (for active) and Fig 2.5 (for inactive)) and may become vascularised (Fig 2.6). They may involve the pars plana for 360°, but are most frequently confined to the inferior fundus. Snowbanks in patients with active pars planitis have poorly defined edges with overlying vitreous snowballs, and the adjacent vitreous is infiltrated with material extending from the surface into the vitreous cavity (see Fig 2.4). In patients with inactive burnt out inflammation snowbanks are well demarcated, flat, chalky white, and do not have surrounding vitreous infiltration (see Fig 2.5). Uncommonly, they can be extensive covering large areas of retina and be associated with severe vitreous opacification

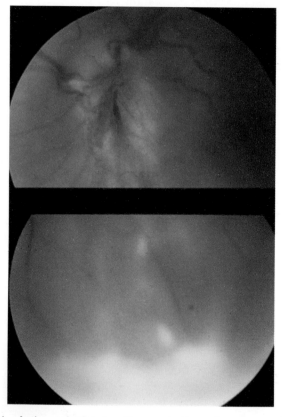

Figure 2.4 Active snowbank with snowballs and new vessels on the optic disc in pars planitis.

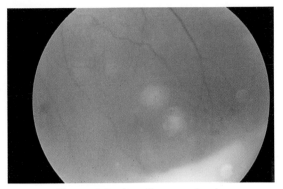

Figure 2.5   Inactive snowbank.

and organisation. Snowbanks may be associated with vitreous traction, retinal detachment, neovascularisation (see Fig 2.6), and the development of retinoschisis (Fig 2.7). The peripheral retina may have irregular retinal pigment epithelial clumping and atrophy and associated retinal atrophy near snowbanks.

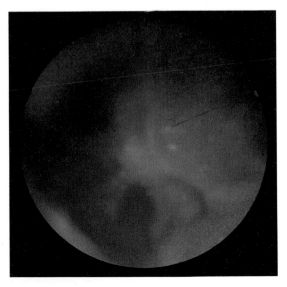

Figure 2.6   Neovascularisation of snowbank.

31

DIFFERENTIAL DIAGNOSIS

The diagnosis of intermediate uveitis is made by identifying the clinical signs of inflammation in the vitreous humour, a lack of focal retinal or choroidal pathology, and the absence of clinical findings that would suggest an alternate ocular diagnosis. There are several common and important systemic diseases that can produce a clinical picture similar to that of idiopathic intermediate uveitis. The most frequent is multiple sclerosis which may produce a range of inflammatory ocular syndromes, including intermediate uveitis. Sarcoidosis, Lyme disease, and syphilis are also able to produce typical intermediate uveitis. Ocular lymphoma should always be considered in adults, particularly in older patients and in those with atypical features. Intermediate uveitis also occurs rarely in patients with Reiter's syndrome, inflammatory bowel disease, and Whipple's disease. Patients with HIV infection may develop a

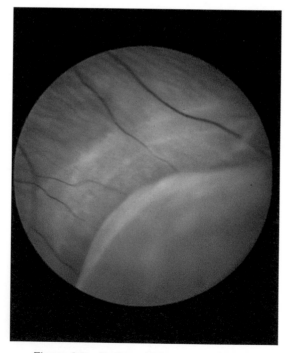

Figure 2.7   Retinoschisis in pars planitis.

Table 2.1   Systemic diseases associated with intermediate uveitis

Disease	Investigations
Multiple sclerosis	MRI, evoked potentials, CSF studies, neurological consultation
Sarcoidosis	Chest radiograph, gallium scanning, MRI, serum ACE level, skin hypersensitivity responses, tissue biopsy, medical consultation
Syphilis	Serology
Lyme disease	Serology
Lymphoma	Vitreous biopsy, CSF studies, MRI CT
Inflammatory bowel disease	Gastroenterology consultation and work-up, biopsies, HLA-B27 determination
Whipple's disease	Serology, medical consultation, and directed investigations and biopsy
Reiter's syndrome	HLA-B27 determination, serology, rheumatology consultation
HIV infection	Serology, vitreous biopsy
HTLV-1 infection	Serology

MRI, magnetic resonance imaging; CSF, cerebrospinal fluid; ACE, angiotensin converting enzyme; CT, computerised tomography.

uveitis similar to intermediate uveitis, as may patients with HTLV-1 infection. A careful review of systems and selective investigations will confirm the underlying disease (Table 2.1).

In unilateral disease, ocular toxocariasis, peripheral retinal toxoplasmosis, and Fuchs' heterochromic cyclitis may develop vitreous changes which closely resemble those of intermediate uveitis. Other diseases that may produce a somewhat similar clinical picture include: amyloid infiltration of vitreous, Coats' disease, and uveitis associated with a retinal tear or detachment (Schwartz's syndrome). In each of these diseases, careful clinical evaluation will allow the correct diagnosis to be made (Table 2.2).

Table 2.2   Ocular diseases associated with intermediate uveitis

Ocular disease	Investigations
Toxocariasis	Serology, local intraocular antibody levels, ultrasonography
Toxoplasmosis	Serology, local intraocular antibody
Fuchs' heterochromic cyclitis	Observation over time, non-response to corticosteroids
Coats' disease	Fluorescein angiography
Amyloidosis	Vitreous biopsy
Schwartz's syndrome	Ultrasonography

Multiple sclerosis

Multiple sclerosis is a progressive, episodic, neurological disease which involves the eye and most commonly produces optic neuritis or gaze disorders. Retinal vascular sheathing (Fig 2.8), retinal vasculitis, chronic anterior uveitis, and intermediate uveitis have each been described in association with multiple sclerosis.[11] Up to 15% of patients with intermediate uveitis will develop multiple sclerosis.[12] There are no ocular features that allow the differentiation of idiopathic intermediate uveitis from that associated with multiple sclerosis. Occasionally ocular disease precedes the onset of neurological disease; however, most patients have had episodes historically which suggest demyelination and there are often subtle neurological signs that will suggest the diagnosis. To recognise such patients, the ophthalmologist must take a careful history for symptoms suggestive of multiple sclerosis, including past episodes of vertigo, ataxia, visual loss, dysphagia, paraesthesiae, weakness, and sphincter dysfunction. A diagnosis of multiple sclerosis has major implications for the patient and must

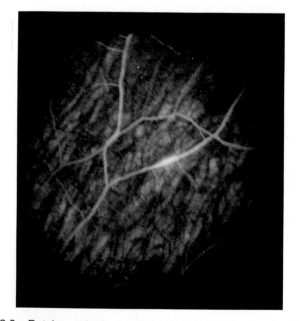

Figure 2.8 Patchy retinal vascular sheathing with localised blood–retinal barrier breakdown, as seen by fluorescein angiography, in multiple sclerosis.

be carefully established. This diagnosis should be established or confirmed by a neurologist. Uveitis associated with multiple sclerosis is managed on its merits, has a similar prognosis to idiopathic disease, and its outcome seems unrelated to that of the neurological disease.

Sarcoidosis

Sarcoidosis is an idiopathic, multisystem, chronic granulomatous inflammatory disease which commonly produces uveitis (see chapter 3). The uveitis may take many forms, including intermediate uveitis, and is most commonly associated with either pulmonary or central nervous system sarcoidosis. A high index of suspicion for sarcoidosis is necessary in all patients with intermediate uveitis, but particularly in patients of Afro-Caribbean descent in whom sarcoidosis is more common. Intermediate uveitis is recognised as a risk factor for a poor visual outcome in patients with ocular sarcoidosis.[13] Rarely, patients with ocular sarcoidosis can develop devastating neurological sarcoidosis which may prove fatal.[14]

Infections

Syphilis must always be excluded in patients with intermediate uveitis as it may produce the clinical picture of intermediate uveitis. More recently, Lyme disease has been shown to cause this clinical picture and, in patients with suggestive clinical features such as erythema chronicum migrans, arthropathy, focal neurological changes, or a history suggestive of exposure, appropriate serology should be performed.[15] Retrovirus infection with either HIV or HTLV-1 may result in intermediate uveitis (Fig 2.9) and appropriate serological testing should be performed when the history is suggestive.[16, 17]

Lymphoma

Intraocular lymphoma must be considered carefully in patients presenting with intermediate uveitis. Traditionally considered to be a disease of older age groups, several studies have shown that it

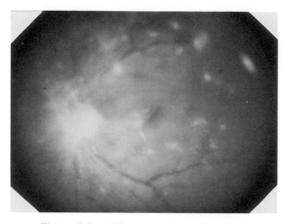

Figure 2.9   HTLV-1 associated uveitis.

occurs in both young and older adults. Rarely, it may be possible to determine clinically that the vitreous cellular infiltrate consists of larger, unusually shaped and clumped cells which are characteristic of those seen in ocular lymphoma. Most commonly, the clinical picture is atypical in that the ocular physical signs are inconsistent. There may be profound vitreous infiltration but little macular or retinal oedema. There may be severe anterior segment changes such as hypopyon uveitis, iris infiltration, and elevated intraocular pressure in the absence of other signs of severe anterior segment inflammation.[18] There also may be retinal (Fig 2.10), subretinal, or choroidal infiltrates (Fig 2.11), and B scan ultrasonographic changes. Neurological symptoms and signs may be present or the patient may have a past history of systemic lymphoma. There may be a poor response to seemingly appropriate therapy. The presence of any of these manifestations should suggest lymphoma as a possible diagnosis and vitreous, endoretinal, or chorioretinal biopsy should be performed to exclude lymphoma. Such patients also require general medical assessment and investigation by neuroimaging studies and lumbar puncture.

MANAGEMENT

The management principles for patients with intermediate uveitis are similar to those for other inflammatory eye diseases (see chapter 8). The first step is to take a thorough history and to perform a detailed ocular examination, including a careful review of systems to look for clues of an associated systemic disease. Investigations are guided by the results of the clinical assessment and review of systems, and the only investigations performed in all patients are a chest radiograph and syphilis serology, because these investigations may significantly alter patient management. Consultation with physicians should be sought for patients who have signs and symptoms that suggest an associated systemic disease such as multiple sclerosis, sarcoidosis, or syphilis.

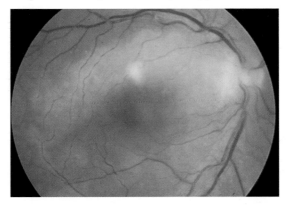

(a)

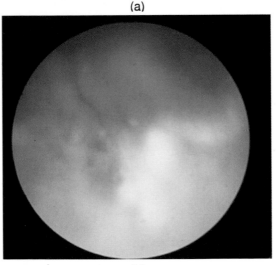

(b)

Figure 2.10   Large cell lymphoma in the retina: (a) a small central white patch; and (b) large area of peripheral retinitis.

37

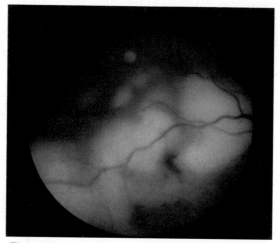

Figure 2.11   Large cell lymphoma in the choroid.

Complications

Complications from intermediate uveitis are frequent and are indications for treatment. Macular oedema with associated reduced visual acuity is the most common indication for treatment. Other common complications include: cataract, elevated intra-ocular pressure and glaucoma, retinal detachment, retinoschisis, epiretinal membrane formation, vitreous haemorrhage, retinal neovascularisation, and cyclitic membrane formation. In a recent retrospective study by Malinowski et al,[12] cataract developed in 80% of patients, macular oedema in 70%, surface wrinkling retinopathy in 44%, and peripheral neovascularisation in 13%. Seventeen per cent of patients developed chronic macular oedema. The management of complications from intermediate uveitis must be individualised according to the complication and the patient.

Outcome

Intermediate uveitis is a common chronic persistent uveitis with a low potential for causing severe visual loss.[19] All patients with intermediate uveitis require a careful clinical assessment, a thorough review of systems, and selective investigations to determine whether there is an underlying or associated systemic disease causing the uveitis. Many patients require no therapy other than observation. Intermittent local therapy is often sufficient to control inflammation, prevent visual loss, and ensure an excellent visual outcome in most patients who do need therapy. In a small number of patients, there is severe disease and a significant threat to vision. These patients may require prolonged, aggressive, immunosuppressive therapy to control inflammation and prevent visual loss. The usual mechanisms of visual loss are chronic macular oedema, cataract, and glaucoma. Patients with pars planitis are particularly susceptible to vitreoretinal complications, including retinal tears, retinal detachment, and epiretinal membrane formation which may result in visual loss. Pars plana vitrectomy may be necessary for the management of these complications, and may also have a therapeutic role earlier in the disease in patients with unilateral disease, or in those who are unresponsive to or cannot tolerate immunosuppressive therapy (see chapter 9).

Intermediate uveitis is a relatively benign disease with a prolonged course which can occur in any age group and which usually results in a good visual outcome even in patients who require systemic immunosuppressive therapy.

1 Bloch-Michel E, Nussenblatt R. International Uveitis Study Group recommendations for the evaluation of intraocular inflammatory disease. *Am J Ophthalmol* 1987;**103**:234–5.
2 Dugel PU, Smith RE. Intermediate uveitis (pars planitis). *Ophthalmol Clin North Am* 1993;**6**:29–37
3 Wetzig R, Chan C-C, Nussenblatt R, et al. Clinical and immunopathological studies of pars planitis in a family. *Br J Ophthalmol* 1988;**72**:5–10.
4 Green WR, Kincaid MC, Michels RG, et al. Pars planitis. *Trans Ophthalmol UK* 1981;**101**:361–9.
5 Yoser SL, Forster DJ, Rao NA. Pathology of intermediate uveitis. *Dev Ophthalmol* 1992;**23**:60–4.
6 Bora NS, Bora PS, Kaplan HJ. Identification, quantification and purification of a 36 kDa circulating protein associated with active pars planitis. *Invest Ophthalmol Vis Sci* 1996;**37**:1870–6.
7 Bora NS, Bora PS, Tandhasetti MT, et al. Molecular cloning sequencing and expression of the 36 kDa circulating protein associated with active pars planitis. *Invest Ophthalmol Vis Sci* 1996;**37**:1877–83.
8 Wistow G. Letters to the Editor. *Invest Ophthalmol Vis Sci* 1996;**37**:2363–4.
9 Malinowski SM, Pulido JS, Goeken NE et al. The association of HLA-B8, B51 and DR2 and multiple sclerosis. *Ophthalmology* 1993;**100**:1199–205.
10 Khodadoust AA, Karnama Y, Stoessel KM, Puklin JE. Pars planitis and autoimmune endotheliopathy. *Am J Ophthalmol* 1986;**102**:633–9.
11 Berger BC, Leopold IH. The incidence of uveitis in multiple sclerosis. *Am J Ophthalmol* 1966;**62**:540–5.
12 Malinowski SM, Pulido JS, Folk JC. Long term visual outcome and complications associated with pars planitis. *Ophthalmology* 1993;**100**:818–26.
13 Dana M, Merayo-Lloves J, Schaumberg DA, Foster CS. Prognosticators for visual outcome in sarcoid uveitis. *Ophthalmology* 1996;**103**:1846–53.

14 Ghabrial R, McCluskey PJ, Wakefield D. The spectrum of sarcoidosis involving the eye and the brain. *Aust N Z J Ophthalmol* 1997; in press.
15 Breeveld J, Rothova A, Kuiper H. Intermediate uveitis and Lyme borreliosis. *Br J Ophthalmol* 1992;**76**:181–2.
16 McCluskey PJ, Hall AJ, Lightman S. HIV related eye disease. *Med J Aust* 1996;**164**:484–6.
17 Mochizuki M, Watanabe T, Yamaguchi K, Tajima K. Human T-Lymphotrophic virus type 1 associated disease. In: *Ocular infection and immunity*, (Pepose JS, Holland GN, Wilhelmus KR, Eds). St Louis, MI: Mosby, 1996.
18 McCluskey PJ, Lightman S. Intermediate uveitis. In: *Inflamaciones Oculares* (Alio J, Ruiz-Moreno J, Carreras B, eds). Barcelona: Edika Med, 1995.
19 Davis JL, Bloch-Michel E. Intermediate uveitis. In: *Ocular infection and immunity* (Pepose JS, Holland GN, Wilhelmus KR, eds). St Louis, MI: Mosby, 1996.

3: Sarcoidosis: systemic and ocular features

Sarcoidosis is a systemic disease characterised by immunological dysfunction with granulomata in multiple organs. Of patients with systemic sarcoidosis 20–30% develop symptomatic ocular involvement at some stage,[1-4] and a significant additional percentage with asymptomatic ocular disease probably remains undetected.[5] A variety of ocular and periocular tissues may be involved, including eyelid skin, orbital, conjunctiva, and intraocular structures, but the uveal tract is the most frequent (>70% of patients), ahead of the lacrimal gland,[1, 2] making sarcoidosis the leading systemic cause of uveitis (3–7% of non-infectious cases).[1, 6] The epidemiology of sarcoidosis varies somewhat according to geographical location. The female preponderance seen in most British studies (1.1–1.7:1) is less than in those from North America (2:1),[7] but in both sexes the disease is most common in the third and fourth decades. The worldwide incidence is higher in individuals of white races than black,[8] but in the USA blacks are affected 15 times more often,[9] and in the UK sarcoidosis is believed to be more common in West Indians[10] and recent young immigrants from Ireland.[11]

CLINICAL FEATURES

Systemic features

Systemic sarcoidosis presents in one third of British patients with the acute onset erythema nodosum–arthropathy–bilateral hilar lymphadenopathy syndrome (EN–arthropathy–BHL). Erythema nodosum is less common (10%) in most North American and other European studies,[8] although the proportion with BHL is high everywhere (70–80%).[10] Hilar lymphadenopathy is unilateral in

3–5% of cases and asymptomatic BHL is discovered in a percentage on routine chest radiography.[12] An onset with either erythema nodosum or asymptomatic BHL is generally of good prognostic significance. The distribution of extra-thoracic organ involvement may be variable in clinical manifestation, but is often much more consistent at a histopathological level. Granulomata are demonstrable on biopsy of the liver, spleen, and skeletal muscle in most patients (about 80%), despite lack of apparent clinical involvement.[13] Cutaneous lesions, such as lupus pernio, are seen in 15% of patients and 15–30% have superficial lymph nodes palpable on examination, especially the supraclavicular nodes, although only a few present because of lymph node or salivary gland enlargement.[7] In addition, 40–50% of patients develop constitutional symptoms including malaise, weight loss, and fever.

Bony changes occur in the phalanges, metacarpals, or metatarsals, and may be associated with swelling and pain on movement of adjacent joints. Skin lesions are often seen in conjunction. Radiologically, the phalanx may be diffusely expanded with a lattice like pattern of rarefaction and overlying swelling and skin changes, but more characteristic most features are localised areas of rarefactions such as bone cysts, usually at the ends of the affected bones, which are often silent clinically.[11] Joint symptoms occur in most patients with erythema nodosum, characterised by an associated transient arthralgia in the large joints of the lower limbs lasting 2–3 months.

In the heart, involvement of the conduction system or the effects of pulmonary hypertension are usually more important than direct granulomatous infiltration of the myocardium. Neurological changes are observed in 5% of patients, usually manifest as a peripheral or cranial neuropathy occurring early in the course of the disease. Involvement of the facial nerve is common, and facial palsy may occur in isolation, or rarely with uveitis and salivary gland enlargement in uveoparotid fever. The palsy is usually transient but 30% are bilateral. Granulomatous inflammation may affect the brain, spinal cord, and meninges, resulting in a prolonged course, but this degree of involvement is usually accompanied by florid manifestations of sarcoidosis elsewhere.

Ocular features

Uveitis is generally an early manifestation, occurring shortly after the appearance of BHL[2, 14] and may adopt one or more of a variety of clinical patterns of inflammatory lesion such as acute and chronic anterior uveitis, vitritis with or without peripheral retinal vasculitis, neovascularisation, isolated or multifocal chorioretinal, or retinal pigment epithelial lesions. Other, non-uveitic lesions such as optic nerve granulomata and occasionally scleritis may occur in isolation.

Anterior uveitis

In about 80% of cases of sarcoid uveitis (60% of all ocular sarcoid) inflammation is limited to the anterior segment,[1, 9, 15] either as an acute anterior uveitis (Fig 3.1), most commonly seen in the acute monophasic type of sarcoidosis together with erythema nodosum and BHL, or as the classic insidious chronic anterior uveitis which is more common in disease of later onset. In this second type, inflammatory Busacca nodules are occasionally seen in the iris stroma (Fig 3.2). The visual prognosis is generally worse in patients with chronic anterior uveitis, with a higher incidence of glaucoma, band keratopathy, and cataract. In addition patients with chronic anterior uveitis may develop clinically significant cystoid macular oedema (CMO), which is rare in the acute form.

Posterior uveitis

The relative incidence of posterior segment disease has been higher in European studies than in American,[4, 16] presumably as a result of differing racial profiles, with a higher proportion of black patients in American studies, but a higher rate of posterior segment

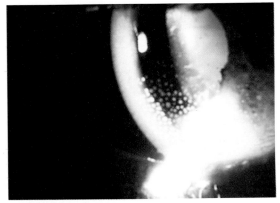

Figure 3.1   Keratic precipitates in sarcoid uveitis.

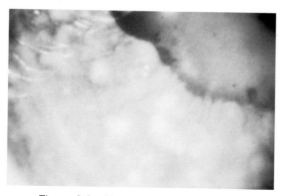

Figure 3.2   Iris nodules in sarcoidosis.

disease in white patients.[4] In the authors' own series the distribution between white (26%) and black (32%) patients was similar, as was the prevalence of posterior uveitis in the two groups (85% and 89%, respectively).[17] Fundus changes usually occur in the presence of some anterior segment inflammation, but this is not invariably the case.[18] In addition, a 35% incidence of central nervous system (CNS) involvement has been reported in patients with posterior segment involvement.[19] In that particular study, however, a disproportionately high proportion of the cases recruited had optic nerve involvement and subsequent reports have not confirmed an association.[20]

Panuveitis

A non-specific anterior uveitis with vitritis is usually seen in association with focal fundus lesions but may also occur in isolation, often complicated by CMO. The vitritis may be characterised by clumping of debris as snowballs or a string of pearls in the inferior vitreous, which may coalesce in the peripheral inferior vitreous giving an appearance similar to the snowbank in pars planitis (see chapter 2).

Retinal vasculitis

Retinal periphlebitis is commonly observed, often just involving small areas of same midperipheral venules. In such cases, severe

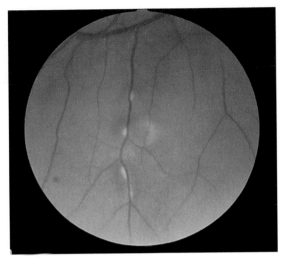

Figure 3.3   Retinal periphlebitis in sarcoidosis.

sequelae are rare. The typical appearance is of a skip lesion with discontinuous areas of sheathing along the venule (Fig 3.3). Severe forms of periphlebitis have been called "candle wax drippings" when large exudates appear to drip from the involved area of vein (Fig 3.4). Subsequent retinal neovascularisation, which may affect the disc or periphery, has been reported in up to 22% of patients,[20] although others have found the incidence to be much lower.[21, 22]

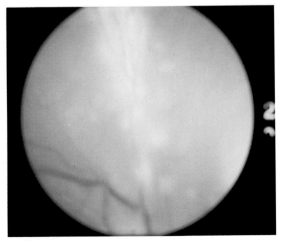

Figure 3.4   "Candle-wax" drippings in sarcoidosis.

Neovascularisation has been reported most frequently in association with areas of closure of small peripheral veins or branch retinal veins as a result of severe periphlebitis.[20] Large vein occlusion is rare.

Choroidal lesions

Multifocal choroiditis (MFC) (Fig 3.2) has been described in the presence of vitritis in a number of reports, distinguishing this as a clinical entity from presumed ocular histoplasmosis syndrome (POHS)[23-27] (see chapter 7) and a proportion is associated with sarcoidosis.[28, 29] Chorioretinitis in association with sarcoidosis (Fig 3.5 and 3.6) was described as long ago as 1925[30] and generally occurs with anterior uveitis and vitritis, although isolated choroidal lesions do occur.[31] The term *"taches de bougie"* was given to these lesions by Franceschetti and Babel in 1949,[32] and is still in use.[19] The term, which means candle wax spots, has not, however, always been differentiated clearly from the candle wax drippings of sarcoidosis associated retinal vasculitis, therefore others have persisted with the term MFC to avoid confusion. These lesions have been identified in anything from 5.5%[21] to 36%[20] of patients with sarcoid uveitis and the visual outcome has been noted to be poorer in these individuals.[16, 29] Two recent studies have examined

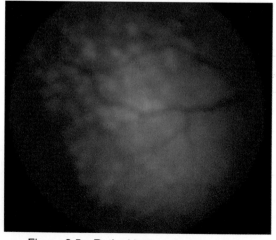

Figure 3.5   Retinal lesions in sarcoidosis.

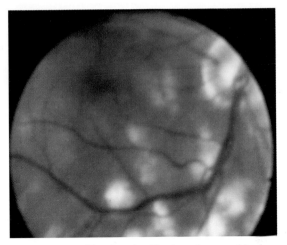

Figure 3.6   Chorioretinal lesions in sarcoidosis.

this type of lesion in sarcoidosis patients.[28, 29] In the first, 7 of 13 eyes with MFC (see chapter 7) and conjunctival biopsies positive for non-caseating granulomata had visual acuities of worse than 20/40.[28] In the second, 22 patients presenting with MFC were subsequently diagnosed as having sarcoidosis.[29] The median age at which the lesions were detected was 52 years in this study, which is similar to that found in the author's own series,[17] and they appear to be more common in older patients with sarcoidosis.

Optic nerve

Although optic nerve granulomata are relatively uncommon,[33] papillitis, neovascularisation, and granulomata of the optic nerve head may occur (Fig 3.7), as well as papilloedema secondary to neurosarcoid. The CNS is involved in about 8% of patients with sarcoidosis and possibly more often in those with posterior segment uveitis.[19, 21]

Other fundus lesions

Other types of fundus lesion such as serpiginous choroiditis have been described occasionally in association with sarcoidosis.

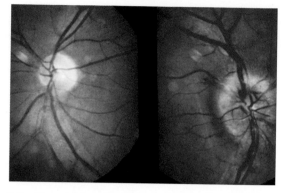

RE   LE

Figure 3.7   Sarcoid granuloma on left optic disc (right is normal).

SYSTEMIC INVESTIGATION

The gold standard for confirmation of the diagnosis of sarcoidosis is the histological demonstration of non-caseating granulomata in involved tissue, in the presence of other clinical features such as BHL on chest radiograph.[34] Certain clinical presentations are, however, highly suggestive of sarcoidosis, including the EN–arthropathy–BHL syndrome. Of particular relevance to ophthalmologists, BHL accompanying uveitis and the rare uveoparotid fever (Heerfordt's syndrome) fall into this category. Isolated asymptomatic BHL is also very suggestive.[11, 35]

Chest radiograph

This is the non-invasive investigation that is likely to yield the most information in the investigation of sarcoidosis. Abnormalities on chest radiographs have been classified according to a simple system of stages 0–III (Table 3.1).[36] Stage I resolves spontaneously

Table 3.1   Staging of Pulmonary Sarcoidosis according to Radiological Findings[36]

Stage	Radiological findings
0	Normal
I	Bilateral hilar lymphadenopathy (BHL) without pulmonary parenchymal involvement
II	BHL with pulmonary parenchymal involvement
III	Pulmonary infiltration without BHL

in 80% of patients, and in 85% of these, radiographic resolution occurs within one year. Pulmonary parenchymal changes tend to be seen in patients with more chronic forms of disease who present at a greater age. Spontaneous resolution occurs in 50–60% of stage II disease and 30% of stage III.[7] In short, spontaneous resolution occurs in two thirds of patients, whereas one third develop a smouldering course. Functional impairment will only occur in 15–20% of all patients.[12] From a diagnostic point of view, the typical parenchymal pulmonary changes are much less specific for sarcoidosis than BHL. In one study of 100 consecutive cases of BHL, 74 were proved subsequently to have sarcoidosis, 20 lymphomas, four lung carcinoma, and two extra-thoracic malignancies.[35] More importantly, however, all 30 asymptomatic patients in this series had sarcoidosis as did all 13 patients with either EN or uveitis. It is therefore debatable whether all patients with asymptomatic BHL require invasive investigations to obtain a tissue diagnosis. It must be emphasised that particular study was performed in 1973 and HIV related thoracic disease, such as lymphoma, may now be an important consideration in the differential diagnosis of asymptomatic BHL. It is important that such patients are assessed by a respiratory physician, especially if systemic corticosteroid therapy is to be instituted.

Angiotensin converting enzyme

Sarcoid granulomata synthesise angiotensin converting enzyme (ACE), and hence serum ACE levels are elevated in about 50% of patients with sarcoidosis overall, and in a higher percentage of patients with active disease. Levels of ACE generally correlate with the activity of disease but are not specific for sarcoidosis and are not usually sensitive enough for screening purposes.[37]

Lysozyme and calcium

Other investigations such as lysozyme and serum or urinary calcium may be helpful. Lysozyme is also produced by the sarcoid granuloma and levels tend to mirror ACE levels, but have a similarly low specificity for sarcoidosis. Ten per cent of patients with tuberculosis have elevated ACE levels but most have elevated lysozyme.[37] The predictive value for serum ACE and lysozyme in the diagnosis of ocular sarcoidosis has been calculated at 47% and 12%, respectively, in one study of 221 patients with uveitis.[38]

Calcium metabolism is disturbed in sarcoidosis as a result of an abnormal sensitivity to vitamin D. This is caused by increased activity of 1,25-dihydroxycholecalciferol ($1,25[OH]D_3$) which is secreted by alveolar macrophages, independent of parathyroid hormone control, resulting in increased gut absorption of calcium and hypercalciuria. Hypercalcaemia is less common.

Pulmonary function testing

Pulmonary function tests may show an obstructive component but a restrictive pattern is more typical.[7] Of patients 40–70% will have a reduction in the forced vital capacity and diffusion capacity for carbon monoxide.

HISTOLOGICAL CONFIRMATION

Histological confirmation may be achieved by biopsy of an obvious skin lesion, enlarged lacrimal or salivary gland, scalene lymph node, or conjunctival nodule if present, but in many cases transbronchial or Kveim biopsy is required.

Conjunctival biopsy

Although conjunctival biopsy may be performed quickly at the slitlamp, its role in the absence of clinical evidence of conjunctival granulomata is controversial. Some believe blind biopsy to be a useful technique[28, 39] but most do not.[5, 37] Biopsy is much more likely to be fruitful where lesions are visible clinically, although in one prospective study a high yield was reported when a 10–12 mm strip of conjunctiva was biopsied.[40]

Kveim test

The Kveim–Siltzbach test is performed using an aqueous suspension of sarcoidosis enlarged spleen. The active ingredient is insoluble, resistant to protease and nuclease digestion, relatively heat stable, but inactivated by alkali. The suspension is injected intradermally and, in reactive individuals, a small papule develops that is most prominent 4–6 weeks after injection. Biopsy of the site is required to confirm the presence of granulomatous inflammation. The proportion of patients with sarcoidosis who are positive is highest in the acute phase with BHL and erythema nodosum (85–90%). With increasing chronicity of disease, the proportion diminishes. Similarly, only 30–40% of those with later onset disease, which tends to be more localised, are positive. Reactivity is proportional to disease activity overall and is suppressed with corticosteroid treatment. Positive reactions have also been described in Crohn's disease, but the main current concern about this technique is the hypothetical risk of disease transmission by injecting human tissue. Consequently, a number of institutions no longer perform Kveim testing.

Transbronchial biopsy

Fibreoptic bronchoscopy with transbronchial biopsy is one of the most sensitive methods of obtaining histological confirmation in sarcoidosis and has been reported to be positive in 60–70% of patients with BHL on chest radiograph and 85–90% with abnormal parenchyma on chest radiograph.[41]

Biopsy of other sites

The relative yields from biopsy of other sites have been tabulated in a review by Jabs.[22]

Lacrimal gland

The value of lacrimal gland biopsy is controversial as a result of the risk of permanent reduction of tear secretion if significant amounts of the palpebral lobe are excised. Using a transconjunctival approach, excision of small amounts of superficial palpebral lobe tissue has been reported to be safe. This technique

51

is probably more useful if the lacrimal glands are clinically enlarged.[42]

Salivary gland biopsy

Biopsy of minor salivary glands in the lower lip can be performed simply using local anaesthesia in the outpatient clinic and has been reported to have an overall yield in the region of 58%,[43] which is lower than transbronchial biopsy and more invasive techniques such as liver biopsy, but higher than blind conjunctival biopsy.

Eyelid lesions

Lupus pernio type lesions of the skin and eyelids are relatively common, especially in patients with later onset sarcoidosis. These may provide tissue confirmation when present.

Scalene lymph nodes

Biopsy of these nodes has been reported to be very sensitive. Others have, however, reported that non-caseating granulomata on scalene node biopsy are less likely to be the result of sarcoidosis than if obtained from a pulmonary biopsy, for example, transbronchial.[44]

ADDITIONAL INVESTIGATIONS

Gallium-67 citrate localisation

Gallium-67 (^{67}Ga) citrate is taken up by activated macrophages in the lung and has been used as a marker of pulmonary inflammation. Increased uptake has been reported in up to 95% of patients with sarcoidosis, but does not appear to be useful in predicting the clinical course.[7] Scanning of the head and neck may demonstrate uptake by lacrimal and salivary glands (panda appearance) and may be useful in the diagnosis of sarcoidosis,[45] although this test is not specific and does not appear to correlate well with clinical involvement of the lacrimal gland.[4] Up to 25% of patients with increased lacrimal uptake of gallium will have no demonstrable evidence of sarcoidosis elsewhere.[37]

Bronchoalveolar lavage

This technique may be of value when transbronchial biopsy is negative. The harvest of lymphocytes is greater from patients with sarcoidosis but the sensitivity is low and lymphocyte levels correlate poorly with disease activity or prognosis. Measurement of CD4 + T lymphocytes may be of greater value.

Complications and outcome

The anterior and posterior uveitis occurring in sarcoidosis are assessed and managed as are other causes of intraocular inflammation (see chapter 8), with systemic therapy adjusted for management of systemic complications such as lung involvement. Some of the ocular lesions described have the potential to cause sight threatening complications, such as glaucoma in patients with chronic anterior uveitis[2, 14] and CMO, neovascularisation, and optic nerve involvement in those with chronic posterior segment disease, which has been reported to carry a poor visual prognosis.[2, 4, 20] In older patients with a more chronic and relapsing course, a worse prognosis has been described than in the younger patient with the acute monophasic pattern of disease.[3, 17, 22] Younger patients and those with isolated anterior uveitis are more likely to have one or two episodes of inflammation without developing chronic problems.[46] In the authors' own series the number of episodes was not examined, but the visual outlook was poorer in patients presenting at a greater age.[17] The worst outcome was seen in those with punched out MFC. The poor visual outcome experienced by that particular group of patients was chiefly the result of glaucoma and chronic CMO. The increased risk of a poor outcome is, however, confounded in these patients by their tendency to present at a greater age.

Cataract and glaucoma are relatively common complications and, although cataract surgery has been shown to be highly successful,[47] glaucoma still carries a poor visual prognosis in patients with chronic ocular sarcoidosis.[2, 21]

1 James DG, Neville E, Langley DA. Ocular sarcoidosis. *Trans Ophthalmol Soc UK* 1976;**96**:133.
2 Jabs DA, Johns CJ. Ocular involvement in chronic sarcoidosis. *Am J Ophthalmol* 1986;**102**:297–301.
3 Karma A, Huhti E, Poukkula A. Course and outcome of ocular sarcoidosis. *Am J Ophthalmol* 1988;**106**:467–72.
4 Rothova A, Alberts C, Glasius E, Kijlstra A, Buitenhuis HJ, Breebaart AC. Risk factors for ocular sarcoidosis. *Doc Ophthalmol* 1989;**72**:287–96.
5 O'Connor GR. Ocular sarcoidosis. *Trans New Orleans Acad Ophthalmol* 1983;**31**:211–22.
6 Rothova A, Bruitenhuz HJ, Meenken L, et al. Uveitis and systemic disease. *Br J Ophthalmol* 1992;**76**:137–41.
7 Weissler JC. Sarcoidosis: immunology and clinical management. *Am J Med Sci* 1994;**307**:233–45.
8 James DG, Neville E, Siltzbach LE, et al. A worldwide review of sarcoidosis. *Ann NY Acad Sci* 1976;**278**:321–34.
9 Mayers M. Ocular sarcoidosis. *Int Ophthalmol Clin* 1990;**30**:257–63.
10 Siltzbach LE, James DG, Neville E, et al. Course and prognosis of sarcoidosis around the world. *Am J Med.* 1974;**57**:847–52.
11 Scadding JG. Possibly infectious diseases: sarcoidosis. In: *Oxford Textbook of Medicine*, 2nd edn (Weatherall DJ, Ledingham JG, Warrell DA, eds). Oxford: Oxford University Press, 1987.
12 Chesnutt AN. Enigmas in sarcoidosis. *West J Med* 1995;**162**:519–26.
13 Johns CJ, Schonfeld SA, Scott PP, Zachary JB, MacGregor MI. Longitudinal study of chronic sarcoidosis with low-dose maintenance corticosteroid therapy. *Ann NY Acad Sci* 1986;**465**:702–10.
14 Iwata K, Nanba K, Sobue K, Abe H. Ocular sarcoidosis: evaluation of intraocular findings. *Ann NY Acad Sci* 1976;**278**:445–54.
15 Ohara K, Okubo A, Sasaki H, Kamata K. Intraocular manifestations of systemic sarcoidosis. *Jpn J Ophthalmol* 1992;**36**:452–7.
16 Bienfait MF, Baarsma GS. Sixteen cases of uveitis associated with sarcoidosis. *Int Ophthalmol* 1986;**9**:243–6.
17 Barton K, Pavesio CE, Towler HMA, DuBois RM, Lightman S. Visual loss in sarcoid-related uveitis. Manuscript submitted..
18 Spalton DJ. Fundus changes in sarcoidosis: review of 33 patients with histological confirmation. *Trans Ophthalmol Soc UK* 1979;**88**:167–9.
19 Gould H, Kaufmann HE. Sarcoid of the fundus. *Arch Ophthalmol* 1961;**65**:453–6.
20 Spalton DJ, Sanders MD. Fundus changes in histologically confirmed sarcoidosis. *Br J Ophthalmol* 1981;**65**:348–58.
21 Obenauf CD, Shaw HE, Sydnor CF, Klintworth GK. Sarcoidosis and its ophthalmic manifestations. *Am J Ophthalmol* 1978;**86**:648–55.
22 Jabs DA. Sarcoidosis. In: *Retina*. (Ryan SJ, ed.) St Louis, MI: Mosby, 1989: 687–95.
23 Nozik RA, Dorsch W. A new chorioretinopathy associated with anterior uveitis. *Am J Ophthalmol* 1973;**76**:758–62.
24 Dreyer RF, Gass JDM. Multifocal choroiditis and panuveitis. *Arch Ophthalmol* 1984;**102**:1776–84.

25 Morgan CM, Schatz H. Recurrent multifocal choroiditis. *Ophthalmology* 1986;**93**:1138–47.
26 Deutsch TA, Tessler HH. Inflammatory pseudohistoplasmosis. *Ann Ophthalmol.* 1985;**17**:461–5.
27 Gass JDM, Margo CE, Levy MH. Progressive subretinal fibrosis and blindness in patients with multifocal granulomatous chorioretinitis. *Am J Ophthalmol* 1996;**122**:76–85.
28 Hershey JM, Pulido JS, Folberg R, Folk JC, Massicotte SJ. Non-caseating conjunctival granulomas in patients with multifocal choroiditis and panuveitis. *Ophthalmology* 1994;**101**:596–601.
29 Vrabec TR, Augsburger JJ, Fischer DH, Belmont JB, Tashayyod D, Isreal HL. Taches de Bougie. *Ophthalmology* 1995;**102**:1712–21.
30 Hudelo, Rabut. Lupoïdes disséminées de Boeck. *Bull Soc Fr Derm Syph* 1925;**32**:108–9.
31 Olk RJ, Lipmann MJ, Cundiff HC, Daniels J. Solitary choroidal mass as the presenting sign in systemic sarcoidosis. *Br J Ophthalmol* 1983;**67**:826–9.
32 Franceschetti A, Babel J. La chorio-rétinite en "taches de bougie," manifestation de la maladie de Besnier–Boeck. *Ophthalmologica* 1949;**118**:701–10.
33 Gass JDM, Olson CL. Sarcoidosis with optic nerve and retinal involvement. *Arch Ophthalmol* 1976;**94**:945–50.
34 Mitchell DN, Scadding JG, Heard BE, Hinson KFW. Sarcoidosis: histopathological definition and clinical diagnosis. *J Clin Pathol* 1977;**30**:395–408.
35 Winterbauer RH, Belic N, Moores KD. A clinical interpretation of bilateral hilar adenopathy. *Ann Intern Med* 1973;**78**:65–71.
36 James DG, Anderson R, Langley D, Ainslie D. Ocular sarcoidosis. *Br J Ophthalmol* 1964;**48**:461–70.
37 Tessler H, Weinreb RN. Laboratory diagnosis of ophthalmic sarcoidosis. *Surv Ophthalmol* 1984;**28**:653–64.
38 Baarsma GS, La Hey E, Glasius E, de Vries J, Kijlstra A. The predictive value of serum angiotensin converting enzyme and lysozyme levels in the diagnosis of ocular sarcoidosis. *Am J Ophthalmol* 1987;**104**:211–7.
39 Karcioglu ZA, Braer R. Conjunctival biopsy in sarcoidosis. *Am J Ophthalmol* 1985;**99**:68–73.
40 Spaide RF, Ward DL. Conjunctival biopsy in the diagnosis of sarcoidosis. *Br J Ophthalmol* 1990;**74**:469–71.
41 Koerner SK, Sakowitz AJ, Appelman RI, Becker NH, Schoenbaum SW. Transbronchial biopsy lung biopsy for the diagnosis of sarcoidosis. *N Engl J Med* 1975;**293**:268–70.
42 Weinreb RN. Diagnosing sarcoidosis by transconjunctival biopsy of the lacrimal gland. *Am J Ophthalmol* 1984;**97**:573–6.
43 Nessan, Jacoway JR. Biopsy of minor salivary glands in the diagnosis of sarcoidosis. *N Engl J Med* 1979;**301**:922–4.
44 Kent DC, Houk VN, Elliot RC, et al. *Am Rev Respir Dis* 1970;**101**:721–7.
45 Karma A, Huti E, Roukonen AO. Assessment of activity of ocular sarcoidosis by gallium scanning. *Br J Ophthalmol* 1987;**71**:361–7.
46 Duker JS. Sarcoidosis of the posterior segment. In: *Clinical decisions in medical retinal disease* (Tasman WS, ed.) St. Louis, MI: Mosby, 1994:348–53.
47 Akova YA, Foster CS. Cataract surgery in patients with sarcoidosis-associated uveitis. *Ophthalmology* 1994;**101**:473–9.

4: Sympathetic ophthalmia

Sympathetic ophthalmia is an uncommon disease characterised by panuveitis after a penetrating eye injury or intraocular surgery, which affects both eyes unless the injured eye has been removed. The inflammation is insidious in onset, occurring most commonly within three months of the traumatic event, and is characterised by a chronic relapsing and remitting course with progressive visual impairment. Mackenzie[1] coined the term "sympathetic ophthalmia" in his original description of the disease in 1830, although the condition was known about in the time of Hippocrates, and eighteenth century veterinarians were well acquainted with methods of preventing sympathetic ophthalmia in valuable animals that had sustained ocular injuries.[2] It is highly likely that Braille lost his sight in childhood from sympathic ophthalmia, an injury to one eye from a leather awl being followed later by the gradual and complete loss of vision in the other eye about two years later. Fuchs described the histological features of sympathetic ophthalmia in 1905[3] in a seminal paper, but the immunopathogenesis of the initiating mechanisms and antigens responsible for it remain elusive, despite great advances in understanding of the inflammatory process. Sympathetic ophthalmia was one of the earliest ocular conditions to be treated with systemic corticosteroids[4] in the 1950s, which dramatically improved the visual prognosis,[5] as the disease until then had almost inevitably resulted in blindness.

Incidence

The true incidence of sympathetic ophthalmia is very difficult to ascertain accurately because it is essentially a clinical diagnosis with no confirmatory laboratory parameters. Mild, self limiting cases certainly do occur which may be overlooked by both the patient and his or her medical attendants. Recent studies have reported an incidence varying from 0.19% after penetrating injuries and 0.007% after intraocular surgery to earlier estimates of 0.54–17.5%, with an average of 2%.[7-10] In general, sympathetic ophthalmia may arise after any ocular injury involving the uvea, particularly when there is incarceration of uveal tissue.

The most common surgical procedures leading to sympathetic ophthalmia include cataract extraction (when it is usually associated with intraoperative complications), iris surgery including iridectomy, simple retinal detachment repair, and vitreoretinal procedures.[11] Sympathetic ophthalmia may also follow non-penetrating ocular intervention such as laser cyclophoto-coagulation and yttrium–aluminium–garnet (YAG) laser cyclo-ablation.[12] After intraocular surgery, the sex distribution of sympathetic ophthalmia is equal in men and women, whereas the trauma related variety shows a male predominance, reflecting the greater incidence of ocular injuries generally in this group. There are no useful genetic markers which can reliably act as a diagnostic tool,[13] such as the association of HLA-A29 with birdshot chorioretinopathy. The age distribution of sympathetic ophthalmia is predominantly triphasic with two major peaks in the first and seventh decades of life, and a lesser peak in the fourth decade.[14]

Although children have been suspected of having a greater propensity for developing sympathetic ophthalmia,[14] this has not been reliably confirmed, and it is likely that its age distribution reflects the population distribution in general, and the differing incidence of ocular trauma and ocular surgery at different ages.

PATHOLOGY

The pathology in the exciting and sympathising eyes is identical,[16] although the histopathological and immunological features of eyes that have been enucleated at the time of presentation of sympathetic ophthalmia differ slightly from eyes removed later in the disease.[17, 18] The characteristic features are of a granulomatous infiltration of uveal tissue, predominantly by lymphocytes and epithelioid cells, with scanty plasma cells and very few neutrophils (Fig 4.1).[17, 19, 20] Early in the disease process, eosinophils can be seen in the inner choroid. The choriocapillaris is characteristically

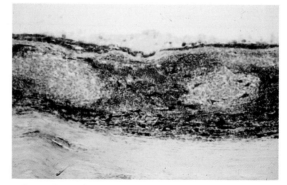

Figure 4.1   Granulomatous inflammation in the choroid in an eye with symphathetic ophthalmia.

not involved but retinal vessels may be cuffed with lymphocytes. Immunohistochemistry of frozen sections has shown that the predominant infiltrating cell is the CD4+ T cell in the early stages of the disease, a proportion of which is activated as shown by their expression of the interleukin 2 (IL-2) receptor. As the disease progresses, more CD8+ T cells are found, but the significance of this is unknown. In experimental autoimmune uveoretinitis (EAU —an experimental model of uveitis), a similar influx of CD8+ T cells is seen later in the disease process, which was proposed as a mechanism of downregulating the inflammatory process. In animals depleted of CD8+ T cells, however, the clinical and histological disease course was exactly the same, making it unlikely that these cells play a major role in this respect. The exact function of the CD8+ T cells in the posterior segment tissues is still elusive, and it is well known that T cell phenotype does not necessarily correlate with in vivo or in vitro function.

Dalén–Fuchs nodules are nodular clusters of epithelioid cells in the choroid and are often pigmented. Retinal pigment epithelial cells may or may not overlie the nodule. Throughout all the inflammatory infiltrate, there is widespread expression of adhesion molecules such as ICAM-1 (intercellular adhesion molecule) and also HLA class II antigens. Although most of the class II antigens are expressed on professional antigen presenting cells, such as macrophages, there is also widespread aberrant expression on cells such as those in the retinal vascular endothelium and retinal pigment epithelium. The stage is therefore set for an autoimmune reaction mediated by T cells to perpetuate the chronic inflammatory process; this process is very similar to that seen in other organ specific autoimmune diseases such as thyroiditis and rheumatoid arthritis. The initiating event is unknown as is the target antigen, but it is likely that, once the inflammatory process has started, many antigens become involved and the perpetuation mechanisms may be largely independent of those that initiated it.

CLINICAL FEATURES

Eighty per cent of patients with sympathetic ophthalmia present within three months and 90% within one year of the traumatic event, with a range reported in the literature varying from 5 days to 66 years.[15] In cases associated with trauma, the peak incidence is usually within 4–8 weeks, but can be longer.

Appropriate treatment may be delayed because of difficulties in establishing a definitive diagnosis, especially when the presentation is atypical or the diagnosis not suspected. The diagnosis of sympathetic ophthalmia must always be considered when a patient develops uveitis in the contralateral eye after surgery or penetrating injury to its fellow, unless there is a previous history of uveitis affecting that eye, or other ocular pathology associated with intraocular inflammation, for example, herpes simplex kerabuveitis, rhegmatogenous retinal detachment, or herpes zoster ophthalmicus.

Although sympathetic ophthalmia is classically described as a panuveitis, anterior uveitis without posterior segment involvement may occasionally occur. Most patients, however, present with a panuveitis of varying severity, ranging from a mild vitritis causing floaters to serous retinal detachments and optic nerve involvement causing a profound reduction in vision. Rarely, a patient may present with advanced visual field loss as a consequence of secondary glaucoma, a frequent complication of sympathetic ophthalmia and a major management problem.

There are no pathognomonic features of the anterior uveitis of sympathetic ophthalmia to alert the physician to the diagnosis, which relies heavily on clinical suspicion. "Mutton fat" keratic precipitates with heavy aqueous flare and a moderate to severe aqueous cellular response are typically present in classic cases, although the keratic precipitates may on occasion be fine or even absent, and the aqueous reaction mild. The intraocular pressure is usually normal at presentation.

59

The extent of posterior segment involvement can be quite variable. Mild cases may show a few posterior vitreous cells, whereas more severe involvement is characterised by disc swelling and serous retinal detachment. Retinal vasculitis and oedema can occur, and the choroid is typically thickened with scattered yellowish lesions (Fig 4.2) which correspond with the histopathological Dalén–Fuchs nodules. Although characteristic of sympathetic ophthalmia, the lesions are not pathognomonic and, in many patients, are not evident until immunosuppressive therapy has been started and posterior segment oedema is resolving. The lesions may become increasingly pigmented (Fig 4.3), which could be so pronounced that it mimics retinitis pigmentosa. Optic nerve involvement characterised by swelling and hyperaemia of the disc may occur, but this is rarely as marked as the intense hyperaemia seen in Vogt–Koyanagi–Harada syndrome (see chapter 17). Choroidal thickening may be most evident on ultrasonography.

Differential diagnosis

The diagnosis of sympathetic ophthalmia is established by careful attention to the history, because the clinical signs are not pathognomonic and may be seen in other types of panuveitis. Once

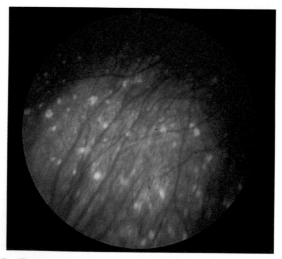

Figure 4.2 Early yellowish Dalén–Fuchs nodules in sympathetic ophthalmia.

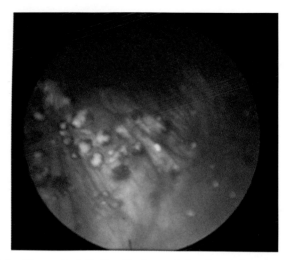

Figure 4.3   Pigmented Dalén–Fuchs nodules in a later stage eye with sympathetic ophthalmia.

a history of trauma or previous ocular surgery has been elicited, there are few differential diagnoses to be considered. In elderly people, intraocular lymphoma should always be suspected, particularly when the degree of vitritis is out of proportion to the visual acuity. Lens induced uveitis may mimic sympathetic ophthalmia and can be distinguished on the characteristic histopathological findings.[16] Vogt–Koyanagi–Harada syndrome and sympathetic ophthalmia share many clinical and immunological features,[21] but are easily distinguished from the history.

Investigations

There is no specific laboratory test that is of help in making this diagnosis. Measurement of lymphocyte transformation to melanin used to be considered specific but is now known to be unhelpful. Enucleation of the injured eye to look for the characteristic histological changes is completely unnecessary, because the clinical signs will be treated on their severity as in any other panuveitis and a specific diagnosis of sympathetic ophthalmia does not alter this. The only useful investigation in the management of sympathetic ophthalmia is a chest radiograph to ensure that there is no tuberculous focus before initiation of steroid therapy.

MANAGEMENT

Not all patients with the diagnosis of sympathetic ophthalmia require systemic treatment. Treatment is necessary for the complications of the disease process only[22] (see chapter 8). Topical steroids and mydriatics are used to suppress anterior uveitis where present and posterior uveitis is treated when sight is threatened or actually impaired. The presence of a few vitreous cells with good visual acuity does not justify treatment, whereas severe vitritis, posterior pole oedema, and serous retinal detachments must be treated aggressively. The systemic therapy of first choice remains corticosteroids and sympathetic ophthalmia usually responds rapidly with regression of the inflammatory signs. As with Vogt–Koyanagi–Harada syndrome, patients with severe inflammatory optic nerve involvement may require higher doses for longer, whereas serous retinal detachments usually resolve rapidly. In some patients, steroids alone are not effective (unusual in sympathetic ophthalmia) or too high a dose is necessary to achieve control (not that uncommon in sympathetic ophthalmia). This necessitates introduction of a second agent, usually cyclosporin A in young patients or azathioprine in older age groups.[23-25]

Occasionally clinically isolated anterior uveitis in sympathetic ophthalmia is not controllable by topical steroids alone and can be extremely severe. These patients are likely to have subclinically active posterior segment disease and will require systemic steroids to quieten the eye.

Complications

Cataract

Phakic patients with sympathetic ophthalmia who require systemic therapy will inevitably develop visually significant cataract necessitating surgical intervention. Intraocular lenses may be safely implanted in these eyes, as long as intraocular inflammation is controlled before surgery and during the postoperative period (see chapter 9). The method of cataract surgery chosen depends on the age of the patient and techniques available to the surgeon. It is imperative to minimise any damage to the conjunctiva during surgery in these patients, because many will subsequently require filtration surgery for secondary glaucoma.

In older children with cataracts secondary to sympathetic ophthalmia, extracapsular cataract surgery or phacoemulsification with insertion of an intraocular lens can usually be undertaken, but if a lens implant is not being considered or the child is very young, then lensectomy with removal of all capsular and cortical remnants can be performed either via the pars plana or by an anterior approach. There is a considerable risk of amblyopia in these younger children, and it is important to implement the appropriate measures, including correction of refractive errors and occlusion therapy, at the earliest opportunity.

Glaucoma

Secondary glaucoma is a significant problem in sympathetic ophthalmia[25, 26] and is usually of open angle type. First line management of glaucoma is with topical therapy (see chapter 8), with reduction of topical corticosteroids to the minimum required to control anterior segment inflammation, because there may be a steroid responsive contribution to the raised pressure. Surgical intervention may be necessary (see chapter 9).

Retinal detachment

Serous retinal detachment may be present at the time of diagnosis of sympathetic ophthalmia and may cause diagnostic difficulties to the unwary, particularly when repair of a rhegmatogenous retinal detachment was the underlying precipitant of the condition. The presence of anterior uveitis should alert the clinician to the possibility of the diagnosis in these circumstances, but this sign cannot always be relied upon to be present. Rhegmatogenous retinal detachment may occur in the sympathising eye as a result of pre-existing risk factors similar to those in the exciting eye or, less commonly, may occur *de novo* as a result of changes in the vitreous and vitreoretinal interface secondary to intraocular inflammation. Serous retinal detachments in sympathetic ophthalmia are highly responsive to treatment with systemic corticosteroids.

Choroidal neovascularisation

As with any type of chorioretinal inflammation, there is an increased risk of the development of choroidal neovascular membranes (CNM), which may arise during periods of inflammatory quiescence. The management of these membranes with laser photocoagulation is similar to that of age related CNM, although, in younger patients, a more expectant policy of observation may be adopted because CNM in this group are said to be less aggressive. Some authorities advocate initial treatment with high dose systemic corticosteroids, and surgical removal of subfoveal CNM may also be considered, but there is a high risk of recurrence, and long term studies of the value of this therapeutic modality are required before this approach can be recommended in this particular group of patients.

Hypotony and phthisis

Hypotony and subsequent phthisis often develop in the exciting eye where it has been retained, although this is by no means inevitable and depends upon the nature of the inciting stimulus. Low intraocular pressure in the sympathising eye at presentation may be secondary to uncontrolled inflammation and may respond to treatment with high dose systemic corticosteroids. A lack of response of the intraocular pressure to corticosteroids often indicates the need for a more intensive approach with an additional agent, such as cyclosporin A. The precarious and unpredictable state of ciliary body function and aqueous outflow facility in these eyes are such that successful control of inflammation may convert a low intraocular pressure at presentation to secondary glaucoma.

The role of enucleation

The management of the exciting eye in sympathetic ophthalmia remains a controversial issue. As a result of the rarity and insidious onset of sympathetic ophthalmia and the frequent delay in recognition of its early manifestations, it is almost impossible to undertake prospective studies of sufficient statistical power to determine the time point at which enucleation after injury ceases to protect the eye from its development. There is, however, no good evidence to support a policy of enucleation once sympathetic ophthalmia is clinically evident, unless for cosmetic reasons or for relief of pain. It can be extremely difficult to assess the visual potential of a severely traumatised eye in the first few weeks after injury, even with the use of electrophysiology, ultrasonography, magnetic resonance imaging, and computed tomography. In particular, the presence of extensive retrohyaloid blood may be associated with profound visual impairment, which may be reversible with the appropriate intervention. If there is "reasonable doubt" regarding the visual potential of an injured eye, then every effort should be made to preserve it because good vision may be retained in an exciting eye, but none when enucleated. Furthermore, a small number of exciting eyes retain a better visual acuity than the sympathising eye, although this will, of course, depend on the nature of the primary insult.

1 Mackenzie W. *A practical treatise on the diseases of the eye*. London: Longmans, 1830.
2 Albert DM, Diaz-Rohena R. A historical review of sympathetic ophthalmia and its epidemiology. *Surv Ophthalmol* 1989;24:1–4.
3 Fuchs E. Über sympathisierende Entzündung (nebst Bemerkungen über sero traumatische Iritis). *Graefes Arch Ophthalmol* 1905;61:365–456.
4 Woods AC. Clinical and experimental observations on the use of ACTH and cortisone in Ocular Inflammatory Disease. *Am J Ophthalmol* 1950;33:1325–49.
5 Reynard M, Riffenburgh RS, Maes EF. Effect of corticosteroid treatment and enucleation on the visual prognosis of sympathetic ophthalmia. *Am J Ophthalmol* 1983;96:290–4.
6 Irvine R. Sympathetic ophthalmia: a clinical review of 63 cases. *Arch Ophthalmol* 1940;24:149–67.
7 Lubin JR, Albert DM, Weinstein M. Sixty-five years of sympathetic ophthalmia: a clinicopathologic review of 105 cases (1913–1978). *Ophthalmology* 1980;87:109–21.
8 Makley TA Jr, Azar A. Sympathetic ophthalmia: a long-term follow-up. *Arch Ophthalmol* 1978;96:257–62.
9 Jennings T, Tessler HH. Twenty cases of sympathetic ophthalmia. *Br J Ophthalmol* 1989;73:140–5.
10 Liddy N, Stuart J. Sympathetic ophthalmia in Canada. *Can J Ophthalmol* 1992;7:552–8.
11 Gass JDM. Sympathetic ophthalmia following vitrectomy. *Am J Ophthalmol* 1982;93:552–8.
12 Lam S, Tessler HH, Lam BL, Wilensky JT. High incidence of sympathetic ophthalmia after contact and noncontact neodymium: YAG cyclotherapy. *Ophthalmology* 1992;99:1818–22.
13 Reynard M, Shulman IA, Azen SP, et al. Histocompatibility antigens in sympathetic ophthalmia. *Am J Ophthalmol* 1983;95:216–21.
14 Duke-Elder S, Perkins ES. Diseases of the uveal tract. In *System of ophthalmology*, vol 9 (Duke-Elder S, ed.). St Louis, MI: 1966, CV Mosby Co, 1966:558–93.
15 Zaharia MA, Lamarche J, Laurin M. Sympathetic uveitis 66 years after injury. *Can J Ophthalmol* 1984;19:240–3.
16 Easom HA, Zimmerman LE. Sympathetic ophthalmia and bilateral phacoanaphylaxis: a clinicopathologic correlation of the sympathogenic and sympathising eyes. *Arch Ophthalmol* 1964;72:9–15.
17 Croxatto JO, Rao NA, McLean IW, Marak GE Jr. Atypical histopathologic features in sympathetic ophthalmia: a study of a hundred cases. *Int Ophthalmol* 1982;4:129–35.
18 Kuppner MC, Liversidge J, McKillop-Smith S, Lumsden L, Forrester JV. Adhesion molecule expression in acute and fibrotic sympathetic ophthalmia. *Curr Eye Res* 1993;12:923–34
19 Jakobiec FA, Marboe CC, Knowles DM III, et al. Human sympathetic ophthalmia: an analysis of the inflammatory infiltrate by hybridoma-monoclonal antibodies. *Ophthalmology* 1983;90:76–95.

20 Kaplan HJ, Waldrep C, Chan WC, et al. Human sympathetic ophthalmia: Immunologic analysis of the vitreous and uvea. *Arch Ophthalmol* 1986;**104**:240–4
21 Rao NA, Marak GE. Sympathetic ophthalmia simulating Vogt–Koyanagi–Harada's disease: a clinicopathologic study of four cases. *Jpn J Ophthalmol* 1983;**27**:506–11.
22 Lightman SL. Uveitis: management. *Lancet* 1991;**338**:1501–4.
23 Nussenblatt RB, Palestine AG, Chan CC. Cyclosporin A therapy in the treatment of intraocular inflammatory disease resistant to systemic corticosteroids and cytotoxic agents. *Am J Ophthalmol* 1983;**96**:275–82.
24 Towler HMA, Whiting PH, Forrester JV. Combination low dose Cyclosporin A and steroid therapy in chronic intraocular inflammation. *Eye* 1990;**4**:514–20.
25 Hakin KN, Pearson RV, Lightman SL. Sympathetic ophthalmia: visual results with modern immunosuppressive therapy. *Eye* 1992;**6**:453–5.
26 Chan CC, Roberge FG, Whitcup SM, Nussenblatt RB. 32 cases of sympathetic ophthalmia: A retrospective study at the National Eye Institute, Bethesda, MD, from 1982 to 1992. *Arch Ophthalmol* 1995;**113**:597–600.

5: Toxoplasmosis and toxocariasis

Toxoplasmosis is caused by a protozoan, *Toxoplasma gondii*, which is an obligate intracellular parasite that can infect warm blooded animals, and also reptiles and fish. It is the most common cause of retinochoroiditis in humans and, even though the causative organism was described at the beginning of the century, the life cycle was only understood in 1970, and most of the aspects related to the interactions between the parasite and the host are still unknown. The formation of tissue cysts, after an acute infection, which shows a predilection for some organs, is still poorly understood. The mechanism for recurrences of the infection, with its most devastating consequences in the eye and the brain, has not been elucidated.

Life cycle

The Felidae are the definitive hosts for *T. gondii*[1] and after primary infection oocysts are shed in the faeces for periods varying from 7 to 20 days with peak production between days 5 and 8.[2] The oocysts are initially unsporulated and thus not immediately infective. After 1–4 days at room temperature, they become infective and may remain so for more than one year in warm, moist soil. Oocysts do not sporulate below 4°C or above 37°C.[3]

Fully sporulated oocysts ingested by intermediate hosts are resistant to the peptic digestion within the stomach, but break down under the effect of trypsin digestion in the small intestine, releasing viable organisms, which are resistant to exposure to the same enzymes for several hours.[2] These organisms are the extracellular forms or tachyzoites which will invade the intestinal mucosa of the host, starting the asexual phase of the life cycle.

Penetration of host cells occurs very rapidly, primarily by active invasion with only a few, probably non-viable, organisms entering by phagocytosis, the mechanism previously proposed by others as the main method of penetration. Inside the cell the organisms will multiply and lead to either rupture of the cell releasing tachyzoites, which will invade new cells, or the formation of a cyst, which represents the "resting" stage of the parasite. *Toxoplasma gondii* cysts are usually subspherical or conform to the shape of the host cell.

PATHOGENISIS
Transmission

Transmission of *Toxoplasma* sp. to humans may occur by direct contact with contaminated soil, by the ingestion of food containing the tissue cysts or vertically through the placenta. In the same way as humans, other animals can also be infected as intermediate hosts and, as a consequence of this, toxoplasma cysts will be formed in their tissues. Ingestion of contaminated meat represents, in this way, an important source of transmission. These cysts are not invariably destroyed by freezing, but will be eliminated by cooking meat to 70°C.[1] Most studies indicate that beef is less frequently contaminated than pork or lamb.[1, 4]

Acquired transmission is probably the most common form of infection, and causes a wide spectrum of presentations, varying from the most frequent of subclinical lymphadenopathy to fulminating pneumonitis and encephalitis, which is probably related to the virulence of different strains and to the immunological competence of the host. Other forms of transmission include blood transfusion from asymptomatic people with parasitaemia, organ transplantation, laboratory accident, and ingestion of untreated cows' milk.

Congenital transmission is believed to result from acute but often subclinical maternal infection acquired during pregnancy.[5] The optimal conditions for transmission are the initial parasitaemia that occurs before development of cellular immunity in the mother and a well developed placental blood flow at the end of pregnancy.[2] Congenital disease may have several different manifestations, including abortion, stillbirth, live born offspring with severe multiple organ involvement, or offspring that are asymptomatic at birth but with neurological and ocular sequelae later in life,[6] depending on the time of infection during pregnancy.[5] The more severe sequelae are related to infection acquired from the second to the sixth months of pregnancy; transmission in the third trimester is more frequent, but usually associated with subclinical disease.[5] It is important to note that infection acquired during pregnancy does not necessarily result in congenital infection and, in subsequent pregnancies after the birth of a child with congenital disease, the maternal humoral antibodies will protect subsequent fetuses from infection.[7]

Chronic infection

After an active infection the disease enters a chronic stage when tissue cysts are formed, mainly in the brain, skeletal muscles, heart, and eyes.[1] In these tissues, cysts will form as early as eight days after infection and they eventually may contain hundreds or thousands of organisms that show slow metabolic activity and are known as bradyzoites. Cysts may persist throughout life without evoking a host tissue response[1,2] or may rupture intermittently causing recurrences of infection.

Ocular disease

Ocular toxoplasmosis has been considered by many authors as primarily a result of congenital infection.[7] Even in the cases where no previous scar is visible in the retina of an adult, the inflammation may result from rupture of cysts present in the nerve fibre layer of the retina since birth. The sporadic attacks of retinochoroiditis may be associated with rupture of tissue cysts,[8] but another theory proposes that the mechanism is related to the development of hypersensitivity to retinal autoantigens.[9] At this moment there is no definitive conclusion about the origin of recurrences, and it is certainly possible that the inflammation is the result of a combination of these mechanisms. The arguments in favour of a congenital origin were based on the fact that few cases of retinochoroiditis have been found in association with active, acquired, systemic disease. Authors have, however, reported cases of retinochoroiditis in patients with acute acquired toxoplasmosis, confirmed by high titres of immunoglobulin M (IgM) detected by indirect immunofluorescence.[10] In one report, eight patients with unilateral focal retinochoroiditis, had positive IgM antibodies against *T. gondii* and seven of them had concurrent high IgG levels.[11] The importance of acquired toxoplasma infection in the pathogenesis of ocular disease was demonstrated by a study that described families, with no twins, in which three to six siblings had documented retinochoroiditis; many of these patients had IgM serum antibodies suggesting a recently acquired infection.[11]

CLINICAL FEATURES

The classic clinical presentation of an active lesion is that of a fluffy, white, elevated focus of necrotising retinochoroiditis (Fig 5.1) near an old scar (satellite lesion) (Figs 5.2 and 5.3). This lesion can vary greatly in size, is usually oval or circular, and more frequently located posterior to the equator. The central, bilateral lesions, especially the macular ones, are more common in the congenital form, although Hogan[12] found that 30% of the congenital lesions were unilateral. The acquired form tends to be unilateral, discrete, and solitary, which makes bilaterality not an essential element in the diagnosis of these lesions. The preference

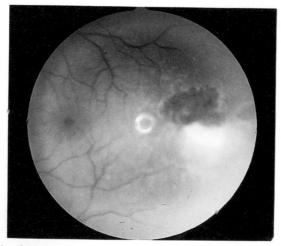

Figure 5.1   Active lesion of toxoplasma chorioretinitis on the edge of an old scar.

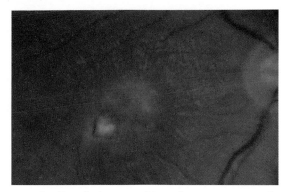

Figure 5.2   Small pigmented toxoplasma scar near fovea.

for the posterior pole, and more specifically for the macula in younger patients, is not clearly understood, but some authors have proposed that it is related to the fact that the organisms gain access to the eye via the optic nerve or posterior ciliary arteries. The lesion classically begins in the superficial layers of the retina, but with progression of the inflammation, the deeper retinal layers, as well as the choroid and sclera, can become involved. There is considerable exudation of cells into the vitreous, particularly overlying the active lesions. When the retina can barely be seen because of vitreous inflammation, an active retinitis can still be glimpsed as a "headlight in the fog". Another subset of clinical

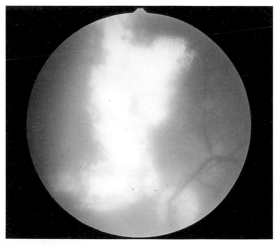

Figure 5.3   Large non-pigmented toxoplasma scar.

presentation, characterised by grey–white fine punctate lesions of the deep retina, with initially little or no overlying vitreal activity, has also been described by some authors.[13] Cases of unilateral pseudoretinitis pigmentosa in eyes with classic toxoplasmosis have recently been described.[14]

A severe anterior uveitis is common with keratic precipitates which may be mutton fat or fine in type and is often associated with a rise in intraocular pressure; this may or may not settle when the inflammation subsides, and cataract formation may occur over a longer time period. This inflammation is assumed to be a hypersensitivity phenomenon, because actual infection of the anterior segment by T. gondii has never been demonstrated in an immunocompetent host.

Direct optic nerve involvement by toxoplasma organisms was first described by Zimmerman,[15] and cases reported as Jensen's juxtapapillary retinochoroiditis, initially specifically associated with tuberculosis, might in fact be caused by toxoplasmosis.[16] A picture of toxoplasmosis neuroretinitis has been described in five patients who developed a sudden decrease in visual acuity with optic nerve oedema, vitreous inflammation, and macular star formation.[17] These patients had positive serology for toxoplasmosis and the features that differentiate this presentation from idiopathic neuroretinitis were the permanent loss of vision in one patient and the presence of recurrent episodes in two patients. Peripheral lesions, probably caused by toxoplasmosis, have also been described, including a wide, ring like lesion near the extreme periphery resembling the snowbanking seen in pars planitis.[18] The incidence of peripheral lesions is very likely to be much higher than the reported rates, which is probably a result of its clinical unimportance. Some authors[19] have described the association of chorioretinal scars typical of toxoplasmosis in cases of Fuchs' heterochromic cyclitis, but a recent study comparing the presence of toxoplasmic scars and non-toxoplasmic scars with Fuchs' cyclitis has shown no statistical significance in the association of toxoplasmic scars and this condition.[20]

Complications

Scleral involvement in toxoplasmosis has recently been emphasised[21] as a more common occurrence than previously thought. Retinal vascular involvement may occur as diffuse or segmental

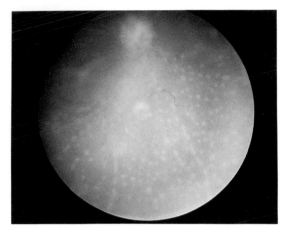

Figure 5.4   Characteristic pattern of vascular sheathing in an active toxoplasma lesion.

perivascular sheathing, involving the vessels in the vicinity of, as well as remote to, a focus of active retinitis[22] (Fig 5.4). The perivasculitis is secondary to a reaction between local antigens and circulating antibody, and the beads seen along the vessels represent cuffs of mononuclear cells. Branch artery obstruction, although infrequent, has been described when a vessel passes through an acute toxoplasmic lesion[23] (Fig 5.5). Choroidal neovascularisation can also be associated with toxoplasmic scars,[24] and may represent

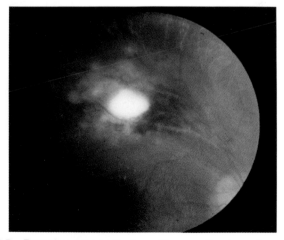

Figure 5.5   Branch artery occlusion with an active toxoplasma lesion.

73

an important cause of visual loss.

Vision may be decreased by vitreous opacification alone, but macular oedema is often observed in the acute or subacute phase of inflammation, and can occur even when the focus of retinitis is located far from it, in a phenomenon similar to that seen in pars planitis.[18] In cases of continuing inflammatory disease, the vitreous humour may contract and lead to posterior vitreous and even retinal detachment. In cases of posterior hyaloid detachment, precipitates of inflammatory cells, the equivalent of keratic precipitates in the anterior segment of the eye, are seen on the posterior face of the vitreous (Fig 5.6).

Immunocompromised hosts

Immunocompromised hosts, either because of immunosuppressive therapy, malignancies, or AIDS, are at high risk for serious disseminated toxoplasmosis. In these individuals recurrent toxoplasmosis represents the most common cause of central nervous system (CNS) mass lesions. Neurological symptoms have been reported in 30–70% of patients with AIDS.[25] Although not as frequently reported as CNS involvement, recurrent retinochoroiditis is found in patients with AIDS.[26] It has been hypothesised

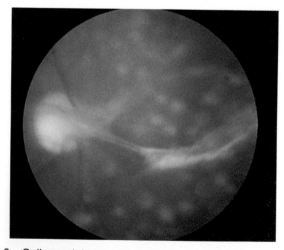

Figure 5.6 Cell precipitates on posterior face of vitreous in active toxoplasmosis with a posterior vitreous detachment.

that only 1–3% of ocular infections in patients with AIDS are caused by *T. gondii*.[27] In one report ocular toxoplasmosis was the first opportunistic infection in 13 HIV positive patients and preceded serological diagnosis of HIV infection in five.[28] There may be several clinical manifestations, including single discrete lesions in one or both eyes, multifocal discrete lesions, or diffuse areas of retinal necrosis.[26] A pattern of bilateral miliary retinitis, initially diagnosed as fungal retinitis, has been described in a 28 year old AIDS patient.[28]

One report describes a unilateral case of diffuse necrotising retinochoroiditis resembling acute retinal necrosis[29] in an AIDS patient. Cases of ocular toxoplasmosis in AIDS patients have been misdiagnosed as panophthalmitis because of the severe intraocular reaction, with the definitive diagnosis being established only by light and electron microscopy.[30] Such a severe form of presentation had been previously reported in association with iatrogenic immunosuppression and lymphoma.[31] The clinical findings in these patients suggest that the ocular lesions result from acquired disease.[26] In AIDS and other immunodeficiency states, the lesions frequently begin adjacent to a retinal blood vessel, suggesting haematogenous spread.[32] The possibility of extension from the brain via the optic nerve has also been considered in some cases.[26] The proliferation of toxoplasma organisms in tissues other than the retina is another important observation in AIDS patients.[32, 33] Histopathological study of two patients has shown extensive retinal necrosis, little inflammation, and the presence of organisms in the retinal pigment epithelium, choroid, and retina.[26]

Investigations

The diagnosis of ocular toxoplasmosis is based primarily on the clinical characteristics of a focal, necrotising retinitis. Several serological tests are available, but as a result of the presence of anti-toxoplasma IgG antibodies in the population (as a consequence of past acquired infection), and also the fact that serum antibody titres are often low in cases where ocular inflammation appears to be the only manifestation of the disease, they have limited application. A negative serological test in undiluted serum does not exclude the infection but makes it highly improbable.[34] On the other hand, a positive test will only be significant in the presence of a compatible ocular lesion.

In cases where the clinical picture is atypical, or the view of the fundus is poor as a result of intense vitritis, or even in cases in which other infectious diseases must be considered, studies of the aqueous and vitreous humour may be helpful. The ratio between local and systemic levels of specific antibodies indicate ocular infection if more antibody per unit of γ-globulin can be detected in the aqueous humour than in the serum.[35] This ratio can be calculated as the Witmer–Goldman coefficient:

$$\frac{\text{antibody titre aqueous}}{\text{total immunoglobulin aqueous}} : \frac{\text{antibody titre serum}}{\text{total immunoglobulin serum}}$$

Values greater than 1 would indicate local production of antibody, but, in practice, the result should be greater than 8 for the diagnosis. The polymerase chain reaction (PCR) has also been successfully used in the diagnosis of ocular toxoplasmosis using samples from both aqueous and vitreous humour.[36, 37]

MANAGEMENT

The indications for initiating therapy are associated primarily with reduction in visual acuity, location of the active lesion, and intensity of inflammatory reaction reflected in the grade of vitritis. The size of a lesion is less important, but larger lesions (> 1–2 disc diameters), even when peripheral, may require therapy when inducing moderate to marked vitritis. In immunocompetent individuals, most of the damage to intraocular structures is related to the intensity of the inflammatory response. For this reason steroids play a major role in controlling this aspect of the reaction. The use of steroids alone could potentially lead to spread of the infection, with consequent loss of vision and, for this reason, anti-toxoplasma drugs must always be added to the steroids, even though there is no evidence that these drugs are actually capable of altering the course of an acute infection. Healing time for the active lesion varies from several weeks to several months.

The combination of pyrimethamine, sulphadiazine, and systemic corticosteroids is the most commonly used.[38] Folinic acid supplementation should always be used with pyrimethamine. Other combinations include the use of other sulphonamides, clindamycin, and tetracyclines. A recent trial comparing the different therapeutic strategies did not show any difference in the duration of inflammatory activity between treated and untreated patients.[39] The only significant finding was the presence of smaller scars in the pyrimethamine treated group of patients. This finding has implications in the indication for therapy, making pyrimethamine the drug of choice for lesions in the macular area. The need for a delay (24–48 hours) in the start of systemic steroid therapy after the start of antimicrobials is controversial and in practice the drugs are given together.[38] Although there are reports of improvement with the use of periocular steroids, this form of therapy should be avoided because there is at least a theoretical risk of exacerbation of the infection.

Physical modalities of treatment, such as laser photocoagulation and cryotherapy, have been used in cases unresponsive to standard treatment or for those patients in whom drug side effects or toxicity preclude continued treatment. Good results have been reported for active lesions, but they are destructive modalities of treatment without definite benefit. Cataract can occur and may need to be removed. The intraocular pressure may rise as a short term problem during active inflammation or may remain high afterwards, necessitating its control either medically or surgically. Pars plana vitrectomy may be useful in cases of persisting vitreous opacity and epiretinal membranes may benefit from surgery (see chapter 9).

Immunosuppressed patients

All lesions should be treated and maintenance therapy used for the duration of immunosuppression.[34] The same antibiotics used in immunocompetent patients can be used in this situation, adjusting for toxicity and allergic reactions but certicosteriods may not be desirable.

Pregnancy

Treatment during pregnancy is a complex subject. In cases of acute acquired toxoplasmosis during pregnancy, the fetus is the main concern and therapy should be carried out under the supervision an obstetrician and neonatologist. Reactivation of head ocular lesions during pregnancy do not put the fetus at risk for congenital transmission, and need for therapy will depend on the maternal ocular picture. The difficulty in the management of these cases comes from the concern of teratogenesis associated with the use of conventional therapy. There is no convincing evidence of the teratogenicity of pyrimethamine, but it is possible that at early stages in pregnancy, folate deficiency induced by pyrimethamine could induce malformations in the human embryo.[40] Other drugs such as sulfadiazine, clindamycin and spiramycin seem to be favoured for treatment during pregnancy.[38] Spiramycin is a macrolide antibiotic that shows high concentration in the placenta, and has been used safely and with some benefit in expectant mothers.

TOXOCARIASIS

Toxocariasis is caused by the ascarid (roundworm) *Toxocara canis*. The link of *Toxocara* sp. with human disease was made in 1952, when the term "visceral larva migrans" was used for the first time to describe a group of three patients presenting with eosinophilia and systemic symptoms who had histopathological evidence of *Toxocara* sp. infection. The initial association of this parasite with ocular disease was established when a granulomatous inflammatory process, with eosinophilic abscesses, similar to those found in other parts of the body in cases of helminthic infection, were found in eyes that had been enucleated for suspected retinoblastoma. Only a few years later it was determined that the nematode found in these cases was the second stage *Toxocara* sp. larva.

Transmission

Toxocariasis is endemic in all dog populations, although it is more common in warmer regions. It has a high prevalence, greater than 80%, in puppies of 2–6 months of age, decreasing to 20% in dogs older than one year.[41] Most of the dogs in the United States of America are infected with *Toxocara canis* as puppies, whereas it is estimated that around 20% of dogs are infected in southern England.[41] Adult dogs are rarely a source of human infection because complete maturation of larvae into mature adults is uncommon. In pregnant bitches there is reactivation of encysted larvae with infection of puppies occurring *in utero*. Puppies can also be infected by larvae in the milk. Both puppies and lactating bitches begin to shed eggs in their faeces about four weeks *post partum*.[41]

Children and adults acquire the infection by the accidental ingestion of eggs which are eliminated in dog faeces.[42] Some infected patients have a history of geophagia or other forms of pica such as ingestion of clay or grass.[41, 42] Seroprevalence varies from 2.6% to 14.6% in places like London and Bedfordshire, to 80% and 92.8% in places with higher exposure.[43]

CLINICAL FEATURES

Humans are not definitive hosts, and infestation with the second or third stage larva causes two diseases: a systemic form called Visceral larva migrans (VLM) and ocular toxocariasis.

Visceral larva migrans

Visceral larva migrans (VLM) is characterised by fever, pallor, hepatosplenomegaly, coughing or wheezing, anorexia, weight loss, marked eosinophilia, and positive serology to *Toxocara* sp. It usually occurs at a younger age (15–30 months) than that for cases of ocular involvement ($7\frac{1}{2}$ years).[44] The association between the larva of *Toxocara canis* and this systemic syndrome was established by Beaver and associates after studying liver biopsies from three patients.[45] This is an acute form which occurs in younger children (mean age of onset of 2 years) and happens in the setting of a large larval load, serving as a massive antigenic stimulus, which induces an intense immune response with marked eosinophilia.[43] The association of VLM and ocular disease is rare. In 106 seropositive children, Ellis and associates did not find any cases of ocular involvement.[46] In another series of 245 cases of ocular toxocariasis, Brown found only five who reported symptoms of VLM.[44]

Ocular toxocariasis

The ocular form is attributed to the presence of the parasite in the ocular tissue. It occurs in cases of infestation by a low larval load, insufficient to stimulate the immune system, allowing the passage of larvae through the liver and into the general circulation, eventually reaching the eye.[43] Eye disease usually occurs in the absence of simultaneous signs and symptoms of VLM.[44] The ocular form is typically unilateral occurring usually in older children ($7\frac{1}{2}$ years), with 80% of the cases occurring below the age of 16.[44] The clinical spectrum of ocular toxocariasis has usually been divided into three major types which can occur separately or together: chorioretinal granuloma of the posterior pole (Fig 5.7), peripheral chorioretinal granuloma (Fig 5.8), and endophthalmitis (diffuse panuveitis). The granulomata are the result of encystment of a

79

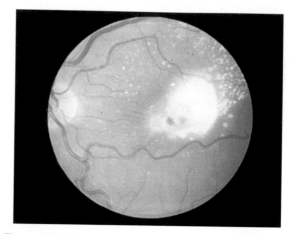

Figure 5.7   Toxocara granuloma at the posterior pole.

second stage larva in the choroid.[47] The frequency of occurrence of these forms is variable depending on the series; some report peripheral lesions as the most frequent form[48] whereas others find posterior disease to be more common.[49]

The posterior pole granuloma is typically unilateral, with an acute stage when a white mass is usually seen, with hard exudates, focal haemorrhages, and, in rare cases, serous retinal detachment. The degree of vitritis in this stage is variable, and when severe may make visualisation of the mass very difficult. In the healing stages

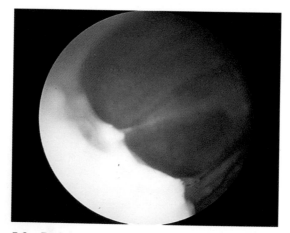
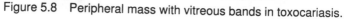

Figure 5.8   Peripheral mass with vitreous bands in toxocariasis.

there is reduction in inflammatory activity, with clearing of haemorrhages and progressive absorption of exudates. In the chronic stage a well defined retinal mass can be seen, with migration of pigment and cicatricial changes in the area surrounding the main lesion. The location of the lesion in the posterior pole is variable, and the size may vary from less than one disc diameter to involvement of the entire macular region.[50]

The peripheral form is caused by an inflammatory reaction which results in the formation of a whitish mass involving the retina and peripheral vitreous (see Fig 5.8). Vitreous membranes are formed and result in the formation of the classic radial retinal falciform folds, which may lead to dragging of the optic disc and macula and in many cases result in poor vision and strabismus. The vitreous membranes can also become organised circumferentially giving the appearance of a snowbank. Very rarely epiretinal membranes will form secondarily in the posterior pole.

The acute stage of endophthalmitis is characterised by inflammation affecting the anterior segment, vitritis, and a yellow–white mass that can be easily misdiagnosed as a retinoblastoma. In the chronic stage a retrolental mass can be seen, with the development of a cyclitic membrane, cataract, glaucoma, and possible progression to phthisis bulbi. Two cases of recurrent panuveitis, without recurrent inflammation in the granulomata, have also been reported, and the authors suggest that this should be considered a different entity in the clinical spectrum of ocular toxocariasis.[51]

Direct optic nerve involvement, although very rare, has been reported by some.[52] Even though cases of anterior segment involvement have been reported, there has been no histological confirmation of such a manifestation.[53]

Diagnosis

The diagnosis of ocular toxocariasis is essentially clinical. Children will present to the ophthalmologist either because of signs of ocular inflammation, including pain, or because of poor vision caused by retinal abnormalities or cataract or its sequelae such as strabismus. A history of contact with puppies of less than three months of age and pica suggest the diagnosis of toxocariasis.[54] In cases where slitlamp biomicroscopy and indirect ophthalmoscopy are not possible, ultrasonography is of considerable value especially where the differential diagnosis is with retinoblastoma, where calcification may be detected (Fig 5.9).

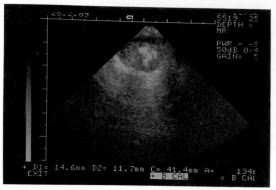

Figure 5.9 Ultrasonography demonstrating calcium in a child with retinoblastoma in whom *Toxocara* sp. was considered to be the cause of the ocular signs.

Investigations

The eosinophil count is not very useful because by the time ocular disease develops, the blood count has usually returned to normal. Tests such as haemagglutination and complement fixation have limited sensitivity as a result of crossreactivity with other anthelminthic antibodies,[50] whereas immunofluorescent antibody techniques using larval secretory antigen are specific but lack sensitivity.[55] The enzyme linked immunosorbent assay (ELISA) test is the most reliable, using two antigens derived from *Toxocara* sp. A titre greater than or equal to 1:16 has been suggested to maximise sensitivity and specificity.[56] In a study looking at prevalence of seropositivity to *Toxocara canis*, the authors found a 31.8% prevalence of seropositivity (titre >1:16) in the absence of ocular toxocariasis, and recommend caution when interpreting seropositivity in cases of possible retinoblastoma that occur in areas of widely prevalent *Toxocara canis* infection.[46] Aspirates from aqueous or vitreous humour allow for both cytological analysis of the predominant cell type involved in the inflammatory process (eosinophils in the case of toxocariasis) and detection of local production of antibodies by the ELISA test.[42]

The definitive diagnosis is only possible by demonstration of the larvae in the ocular tissues.

Differential diagnosis

The differential diagnosis of ocular toxocariasis includes retino-blastoma, Coats' disease, persistent hyperplastic primary vitreous

(PHPV), retinopathy of prematurity (ROP), and pars planitis. In a series from the Wills Eye Hospital, (Philadelphia, USA) from 500 children referred with a diagnosis of possible retinoblastoma, only 288 (58%) had retinoblastoma. Of the 212 (42%) lesions simulating retinoblastoma, presumed ocular toxocariasis was responsible for 16%.[57] Children with retinoblastoma are usually younger and there may be a history of retinoblastoma in the family. In the chronic stages of toxocariasis, the vitreous is usually clear with the presence of vitreoretinal membranes, although the subretinal space is clear. Vitreous and subretinal space involvement in retinoblastoma depends on the endophytic or exophytic growth of the tumour. B scan ultrasonography and computed tomography may show the presence of a calcified mass, and in more difficult cases aqueous cytology and enzymes may be helpful.[42]

Retinal detachment in Coats' disease is clearly exudative, with the peripheral retinal vasculature showing the typical telangiectatic changes. The condition of PHPV is congenital, usually associated with microphthalmos, a retrolenticular mass, and cataract. In ROP the condition is bilateral, with the presence of peripheral microvascular disease and a history of prematurity. Pars planitis also tends to be a bilateral condition, even though some cases may be extremely asymmetrical at presentation. The presence of snowbanking is very characteristic and the degree of vitreous involvement is variable (see chapter 3).

MANAGEMENT

The damage to ocular structures in this condition depends on the location of the primary lesion and the intensity of the secondary inflammatory activity elicited. Topical steroids are very useful in the management of anterior segment inflammation and periocular injection of long acting depot steroids is a good option in cases of mild inflammation of the posterior segment. In cases of severe and diffuse inflammation, systemic corticosteroids are necessary.

The use of antihelminthic agents is controversial because death of the parasite itself can induce significant inflammation, necessitating the use of steroids.[58] As no controlled series are available it is possible that the changes observed during antihelminthic therapy may represent only the natural course of the disease.[41, 42] Laser treatment may be attempted when the larvae are at least 3 mm from the foveola, but this may also produce an inflammatory reaction requiring steroid therapy.[42, 58]

Complications

Vitrectomy may be necessary to release vitreous traction and repair tractional or rhegmatogenous retinal detachments. Cataract may occur, requiring removal for visual improvement, and strabismus may become a cosmetic problem in an eye with poor vision.

Outcome

Visual prognosis is dependent on the severity and location of the anatomical changes (see above).

1 Dubey JP, Beattie CP. *Toxoplasmosis of animals and man.* Boca Raton, FL: CRC Press, 1988:213P.
2 Remington JS, Desmonts G. Toxoplasmosis. In: *Infectious diseases of the fetus and newborn infant* (Remington JS, Klein JD, eds). Philadelphia: Saunders, 1990:90–195.
3 Dubey JP, Miller NL, Frenkel JK. The Toxoplasma gondii oocyst from cat feces. *J Exp Med* 1970;**132**:636–62.
4 Jacobs L, Remington JS, Melton ML. A survey of meat samples from swine, cattle, and sheep for the presence of encysted *Toxoplasma. J Parasitol* 1960;**46**:23–8.
5 Desmonts G, Couvrer J. Toxoplasmosis in pregnancy and its transmission to the fetus. *Bull NY Acad Med* 1974;**50**:146–59.
6 Desmonts G, Couvrer J. Congenital toxoplasmosis. A prospective study of 378 pregnancies. *N Engl J Med* 1974;**290**:1110–16.
7 Perkins ES. Ocular toxoplasmosis. *Br J Ophthalmol* 1973;**57**:1–17.
8 Frenkel JK, Escajadillo A. Cyst rupture as a pathogenic mechanism of toxoplasmic encephalitis. *Am J Trop Med Hyg* 1987;**36**:517–22.
9 Nussenblatt RB, Gery I, Ballintine EJ. Cellular immune responsiveness of uveitis patients to retinal S-antigen. *Am J Ophthalmol* 1980;**89**:173–9.
10 Gump DW, Holden RA. Acquired chorioretinitis due to toxoplasmosis. *Ann Intern Med* 1979;**90**:58–60.
11 Silveira CM, Belfort Jr R, Burnier Jr MNN, Nussenblatt R. Acquired toxoplasmic infection as the cause of toxoplasmic retinochoroiditis in families. *Am J Ophthalmol* 1988;**106**:362–4.
12 Hogan MJ. Ocular toxoplasmosis. *Am J Ophthalmol* 1958;**46**:467–94.
13 Doft BH, Gass DM. Punctate outer retinal toxoplasmosis. *Arch Ophthalmol* 1985;**103**:1332–6.
14 Silveira CM, Belfort Jr R, Nussenblatt R, Farah M, Takahashi W, Imamura P, Burnier Jr M. Unilateral pigmentary retinopathy associated with ocular toxoplasmosis. *Am J Ophthalmol* 1989;**107**:682–4.

15 Zimmerman LE. Diseases of the optic nerve: pathology of demyelinating diseases. *Trans Am Acad Ophth* 1956;60:46–58.

16 Smith RE, Nozik RA. *Uveitis: a clinical approach to diagnosis and management.* Baltimore, MA: Williams & Wilkins, 1990:266P.

17 Fish RH, Hoskins JC, Kline LB. Toxoplasmosis neuroretinitis. *Ophthalmology* 1993;100:1177–82.

18 Nussenblatt RB, Withcup SM, Palestine AG. *Uveitis: Fundamentals and clinical practice.* Chicago: Year Book Medical Publisher, 1996:215.

19 Abreu MT, Belfort Jr R, Hirata PS. Fuchs' heterochromic cyclitis and ocular toxoplasmosis. *Am J Ophthalmol* 1982;93:739–44.

20 La Hey E, Rothova A, Baarsma GS, de Vries J, van Knapen F, Kijlstra A. Fuchs' heterochromic iridocyclitis is not associated with ocular toxoplasmosis. *Arch Ophthalmol* 1992;110:806–11.

21 Schuman JS, Weinberg RS, Ferry AP, Guerry RK. Toxoplasmic scleritis. *Ophthalmology* 1988;95:1399–403.

22 Wise GN, Dollery CT, Henkind P. Segmental retinal periarteritis. *Am J Ophthalmol* 1971;72:210.

23 Morgan CM, Gragoudas ES. Branch artery occlusion associated with recurrent toxoplasmic retinochoroiditis. *Arch Ophthalmol* 1987;105:130–1.

24 Fine SL, Owens SL, Haller JA. Choroidal neovascularization as a late complication of ocular toxoplasmosis. *Am J Ophthalmol* 1981;91:318–22.

25 Snider WD, Simpson DM, Nielsen S, Gold JW, Metroka CE, Posner JB. Neurological complications of acquired immune deficiency syndrome: analysis of 50 patients. *Ann Neurol* 1983;14:403–18.

26 Holland GN, Engstron RE Jr, Glasgow BJ, et al. Ocular toxoplasmosis in patients with the acquired immunodeficiency syndrome. *Am J Ophthalmol* 1988;106:653–67

27 Holland GN. Ophthalmic disorders associated with the acquired immunodeficiency syndrome. In: *AIDS and other sexually transmitted diseases and the eye* (Insler MS, ed.). Orlando, FL: Grune & Stratton, 1987:145–72.

28 Berger BB, Egwuagu CE, Freeman WR, Wiley CA. Miliary toxoplasmic retinitis in acquired immunodeficiency syndrome. *Arch Ophthalmol* 1993;111:373–6.

29 Parke DW, Font RL. Diffuse toxoplasmic retinochoroiditis in a patient with AIDS. *Arch Ophthalmol* 1986;104:571–5.

30 Moorthy RS, Smith RE, Rao NA. Progressive ocular toxoplasmosis in patients with acquired immunodeficiency syndrome. *Am J Ophthalmol* 1993;115:742–7.

31 Yeo JH, Jakobiec FA, Iwamoto T. Opportunistic toxoplasmic retinochoroiditis following chemotherapy for systemic lymphoma. A light and electron microscopic study. *Ophthalmology* 1983;90:885–98.

32 Holland GN. Ocular toxoplasmosis in the immunocompromised host. *Int Ophthalmol* 1989;13:399–402.

33 Rehder JR, Burnier MB Jr., Pavesio CE, Kim MK, Rigueiro M, Petrilli AMN, Belfort R Jr. Acute unilateral toxoplasmic iridocyclitis in an AIDS patient. *Am J Ophthalmol* 1988;106:740–1.

34 Rothova A. Ocular involvement in toxoplasmosis. *Br J Ophthalmol* 1993;77:371–7.

35 Baarsma GS, Luyendijk L, Kijlstra A, et al. Analysis of local antibody production in vitreous humor of patients with severe uveitis. *Am J Ophthalmol* 1991;112:147–50.

36 Manners RM, O,Connell S, Guy EC, Joynson DH, Canning CR, Etchells DE. Use of the polymerase chain reaction in the diagnosis of acquired ocular toxoplasmosis in an immunocompetent adult. *Br J Ophthalmol* 1994;78:583–4.

37 Chan CC, Palestine AG, Li Q, Nussenblatt RB. Diagnosis of ocular toxoplasmosis by the use of immunocytology and the polymerase chain reaction (letter). *Am J Ophthalmol* 1994;117:803–5.

38 Engstrom Jr RE, Holland GN, Nussenblatt RB, Jabs DA. Current practices in

the management of ocular toxoplasmosis. *Am J Ophthalmol* 1991;**111**:601–10.

39 Rothova A, Meenken C, Buitenhuis HJ, et al. Therapy for ocular toxoplasmosis. *Am J Ophthalmol* 1993;**115**:517–23.

40 Harpey JP, Darbois Y, Lefebre G. Teratogenicity of pyrimethamine. *Lancet* 1983;**ii**:399.

41 Schantz PM, Glickman LT. Current concepts in parasitology—Toxocaral visceral larval migrans. *N Engl J Med* 1978;**298**:436–9.

42 Shields JA. Ocular toxocariasis: A review. *Surv Ophthalmol* 1984;**28**:361–81.

43 Glickman LT, Schantz PM. Epidemiology and pathogenesis of zoonotic toxocariasis. *Epidemiol Rev* 1981;**3**:230–50.

44 Brown DH. Ocular *Toxocara canis* II. Clinical review. *J Pediatr Ophthalmol* 1970;**7**:182–91.

45 Beaver PC, Snyder CH, Carrera GM, et al. Chronic eosinophilia due to visceral larva migrans. *Pediatrics* 1952;**4**:7–19.

46 Ellis GS, Pakalnis VA, Worley G, Green JA, Frothingham TE, Sturner RA, Walls KW. *Toxocara canis* infestation. Clinical and epidemiological associations with seropositivity in kindergarten children. *Ophthalmology* 1986;**93**:1032–7.

47 Upadhyay MP, Rai NC. Toxocara granuloma of the retina. *Jpn J Ophthalmol* 1980;**24**:278–81.

48 Wilkinson CP, Welch RB. Intraocular *Toxocara. Am J Ophthalmol* 1971;**71**:921–30.

49 Hagler WH, Pollard ZF, Jarrett WH, et al. Results of surgery for ocular *Toxocara canis. Ophthalmology* 1981;**88**:1081–6.

50 Parke II DW, Shaver RP. Toxocariasis. In: *Ocular infection and immunity,* 1st edn (Pepose JS, Holland GN, Wilhemus KR, eds). St Louis, MI: Mosby, 1996:1225–35.

51 Rowson NJ, Stavrou P, Murray PI. Ocular toxocariasis (letter). *Eye* 1993;**7**:810.

52 Bird AC, Smith JL, Curtin VT. Nematode optic neuritis. *Am J Ophthalmol* 1970;**69**:72–7.

53 Baldone JA, Clark WB, Jung RC. Nematode ophthalmitis: report of two cases. *Am J Ophthalmol* 1964;**57**:763–6.

54 Schantz PM, Meyer D, Glickman LT. Clinical, serologic, and epidemiologic characteristics of ocular toxocariasis. *Am J Trop Med Hyg* 1979;**28**:24–8.

55 Glickman LT, Schantz PM, Dombroske R, et al. Evaluation of serological test for visceral larva migrans. *Am J Trop Med Hyg* 1978;**27**:492–8.

56 Pollard ZF, Jarrett WH, Hagler WS, et al. ELISA for diagnosis of ocular toxocariasis. *Ophthalmology* 1979;**86**:743–9.

57 Shields JA, Parsons HM, Shields CL, Shah P. Lesions simulating retino-blastoma. *J Ped Ophthalmol Strab* 1991;**28**:338–40.

58 Nussenblatt RB, Whitcup SM, Palestine AG. *Toxocara canis* infection. In: *Uveitis —fundamentals and clinical practice.* 2nd edn (Nussenblatt RB, Palestine AG, eds). Chicago: Year Book, 1996:238–43.

6: Behçet's disease and the eye

Behçet's disease is a multisystem, inflammatory disorder of unknown aetiology with serious systemic and ocular manifestations, particularly affecting young adults. The classic triad of uveitis and oral and genital ulcers was described over 50 years ago by Hulusi Behçet,[1] a Turkish dermatologist, although the significance of this cluster of clinical signs had been previously observed by Hippocrates[2] and Adamantiadis.[3] In comparison with other types of retinal vasculitis, Behçet's disease appears to run a more aggressive course, with more frequent and severe recurrences, and has a much poorer prognosis for retention of useful vision in the long term.[4] Despite major advances in the drug therapy of immune mediated diseases since Behçet's original description in 1938, the long term visual prognosis in Behçet's disease remains poor.[5]

Definition

A variety of criteria have been used to distinguish Behçet's disease from other systemic vasculitides, of which two are currently in worldwide use. The International Study Group for Behçet's disease has published its widely used diagnostic criteria[6] (Table 6.1), although, in Japan and some other countries, clinicians prefer to use an earlier classification[7] more akin to Behçet's original description (Table 6.2).

The purpose of defining these criteria has been to facilitate study into the aetiology and treatment of the disease, on both a national and an international basis and, although there is now an enormous amount of literature available on the subject, Behçet's disease

Table 6.1 International Study Group for Behçet's disease: Criteria for diagnosis of Behçet's disease[6]

Recurrent oral ulceration

Plus **TWO** of:
- Recurrent genital ulceration
- Eye lesions:
  - anterior uveitis
  - vitritis
  - posterior uveitis
  - retinal vasculitis

- Skin lesions

  - erythema nodosum
  - pseudofolliculitis
  - papulopustular lesions
  - acneform lesions

- Positive pathergy test

---

remains a clinical enigma. The necessity for revision of the criteria demonstrates that these are, unfortunately, imperfect. Behçet's disease is a clinical diagnosis with no absolutely confirmatory laboratory tests and, although the diagnostic criteria in Tables 6.1 and 6.2 are valuable in clinical research protocols, they may be unhelpful in everyday management.

Table 6.2 Behçet's disease: guide to diagnosis of Behçet's disease

---

Major criteria
Ocular lesions (iridocyclitis, chorioretinitis, and their sequelae)
Recurrent aphthous ulceration of the oral mucosa
Genital ulcers
Skin lesions (erythema nodosum like, thrombophlebitis, folliculitis, cutaneous hypersensitivity)

Minor criteria
Arthritis
Gastroenteritis
Epididymitis
Vascular symptoms
Neuropsychiatric involvement

Types of Behçet's disease
- Complete: all four major criteria simultaneously or at different times, or three major symptoms simultaneously or at different times
- Incomplete: ocular lesion and one major or three minor criteria
- Suspect: two main symptoms simultaneously or at different times
- Possible: one main symptom during clinical course

Epidemiology

Behçet's disease shows a racial predilection, being most common in Japan and the Middle East, and ethnic origin may be a factor contributing to the variable patterns of disease and severity throughout the world. Men are more commonly affected than women, the sex ratio varying from around 3:1 in the United Kingdom to 6:1 in the Middle East and Japan, although the clinical manifestations vary in their expression between the sexes, with mucocutaneous disease being more common in women. Ocular involvement occurs in about 75% of patients with Behçet's disease.[8] In Japan, 20% of all blindness in young and middle aged adults is caused by Behçet's disease.

IMMUNOPATHOLOGY

The immunological predisposition to Behçet's disease was reported by Ohno and colleagues[9] who first documented the association of HLA-B5 in Japan in 1973. Further studies by this group have shown that the primary association is with HLA-B51,[10] and more specifically the allele B*5101. This close association with HLA-B51 has been confirmed in other countries which have a high incidence of Behçet's disease, for example the Middle East, but has not been evident in Western countries where HLA-B5 and HLA-B51 are uncommon, although Kilmartin et al.[11] recently observed a significantly increased incidence of HLA-B51 in a study of 24 native Irish patients with Behçet's disease. The underlying pathogenic mechanisms of the association with HLA-B51 are unknown, but are considered to be related to differences in molecular control of the immune response, although whether this results directly from HLA-B51 or an adjacent gene in the vicinity of the tumour necrosis factor β (TNF-β)gene[12] is uncertain. Although there is a clear statistical association of HLA-B51 with Behçet's disease, the relative risk of disease development is only six to seven times that of controls, in comparison to the 200-fold risk of birdshot choroidopathy in association with HLA-A29.[13] In addition, HLA-B51 is not associated with any particular pattern of ophthalmic involvement or a worse visual prognosis. For these reasons, routine HLA testing has no diagnostic or therapeutic value in the management of Behçet's disease at the moment.

Environmental factors have been considered to contribute to the development of Behçet's disease in susceptible individuals, and infection with *Streptococcus sanguis* has attracted considerable interest, particularly in Japan where hyperreactivity of leucocytes and platelets to *Strep. sanguis* infection has been observed.[14]

Some clinical features of Behçet's disease, such as hypopyon uveitis and pathergy, clearly show that the polymorph is involved in the manifestations of the early stages of the disease. These observations have been cited in support of an infectious aetiology, and were also instrumental in the choice of colchicine therapy.[15] More recent immunohistochemical studies of postmortem eyes in Behçet's disease[16] have confirmed the presence of activated CD4+ T cells and aberrant HLA-DR (class II) expression in retinal vessels, confirming the immune mediated basis of the disease and the rationale for immunosuppressive and immuno-modulatory therapy.

CLINICAL FEATURES
Ocular disease

The clinical ocular features of Behçet's disease are not pathognomonic, but the rapidity and severity of the episodes of intraocular inflammation and the association with characteristic systemic features help to distinguish it from many other patterns of uveitis. The development of a severe non-infectious uveitis should alert the clinician to the possibility of Behçet's disease, and a careful systematic enquiry undertaken. The inflammation may be confined to one compartment of the eye, or the entire uveal tract may be involved. The disease may be unilateral or bilateral at presentation, and eventually involves both eyes in around 95% of patients.[17]

Typically there is a severe anterior uveitis with small, white, non-pigmented keratic precipitates, and a hypopyon may be evident although the incidence of this varies. Hypopyon is more common in patients of Middle Eastern or Japanese extraction, occurring in a quarter to one third of cases, but is seen less frequently (about 10%) in white European patients. Iris nodules are very uncommon which reflects the rapid tempo of the inflammatory process in Behçet's disease.

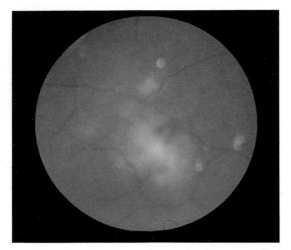

Figure 6.1 Retinal infiltration (white areas) and retinal vasculitis (sheathed vessel) in Behçet's disease. Note the overlying vitreous haze caused by vitritis.

Vitreous inflammation is common, and is most severe when the posterior segment is also involved. Clumps of cells may be present in the vitreous ("snowballs") and, if severe, vitreous opacification may preclude visualisation of the fundus. Degenerative changes in the vitreous arising from recurrent inflammatory episodes lead to premature posterior vitreous detachment, which may be associated

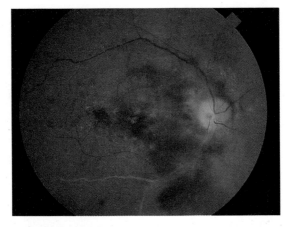

Figure 6.2 Acute occlusive vasculitis in Behçet's disease: retinal oedema and haemorrhage involving the macula with closure of the inferotemporal retinal branch vein.

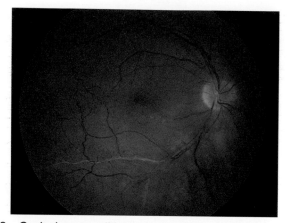

Figure 6.3 Occlusive vasculitis: in the healing phase (compare with Fig 6.2) with recovery of visual acuity to 6/9.

with vitreous haemorrhage either in isolation or secondary to retinal neovascularisation or a retinal tear. Rhegmatogenous and tractional retinal detachment occur in around 5% of eyes.

Retinal involvement is characterised by retinal vasculitis and retinal infiltration (Fig 6.1). The vasculitis may be occlusive or non-occlusive, and is predominantly venous, that is, a phlebitis,

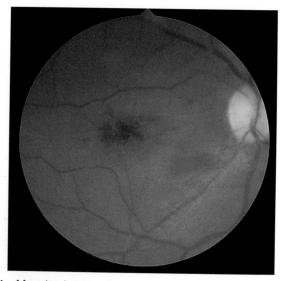

Figure 6.4 Macular haemorrhage and retinal oedema reducing visual acuity to 6/60.

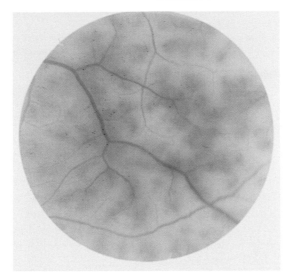

Figure 6.5 Fluorescein angiography in Behçet's disease showing leakage from small vessels (hyperfluorescent areas).

although retinal arterial occlusion is well documented. The presence of multiple areas of peripheral retinal vascular occlusion is highly suggestive of Behçet's disease. Retinal vascular occlusion may be extensive involving a quadrant or more of the retina (Figs 6.2 and 6.3), and can lead to retinal or, rarely, iris neovascularisation.

Macular involvement is a major cause of visual impairment in Behçet's disease. This may be caused by macular oedema, macular

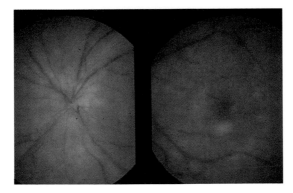

Figure 6.6 Disc swelling and macular retinitis in acute retinal vasculitis in Behçet's disease.

ischaemia (Fig 6.4),[18] or rarely as a result of macular hole formation. Fluorescein angiography may be required to assess the relative contribution from oedema and ischaemia (Fig 6.5). The macula may also be compromised by the development of epiretinal membranes or subretinal neovascularisation.

Disc swelling is common and may occur when there is active retinal vasculitis (Fig 6.6) or direct involvement of the optic nerve, when it is usually associated with visual impairment. Bilateral disc swelling may also, however, result from papilloedema secondary to dural sinus thrombosis, and the finding of disc swelling in the absence of other signs of active intraocular inflammation and normal visual acuity should alert the clinician to this rare complication.[19] Optic atrophy is a frequent sequel to repeated inflammatory episodes, and is a common finding in patients with long standing disease. Disc and retinal neovascularisation as a result of retinal ischaemia are uncommon but well documented, occurring in less than 5% of eyes.

Systemic disease

Oral ulcers

By definition, all patients with Behçet's disease have mouth ulcers. The mouth ulcers of Behçet's disease may be clinically indistinguishable from conventional recurrent oral aphthous ulcers, although they tend to be more painful, extensive, and more frequently involve the soft palate and oropharynx.[20] Oral ulceration may be very severe and distressing, and this has led to the revival of thalidomide[21] as a therapeutic agent, for which it can be very effective.

Genital ulcers

These are less common than oral ulcers, but typically are painful and may involve the scrotum and penis, or vulva.

Skin lesions

Cutaneous involvement includes erythema nodosum, superficial thrombophlebitis, and pustular skin eruptions. The pathergy test is the delayed development (24–36 hours) of a pustule at the site of an intradermal needle puncture which occasionally the observant patient may have noted after venepuncture.

Joints

The arthropathy of Behçet's disease is non-specific synovitis without joint destruction, tending to involve the larger joints, although any joint may be affected.

Central nervous system

Central nervous system involvement may occur and present with brainstem signs, meningoencephalitis, or confusional states either in isolation or as a combination of the three, and is associated with increased mortality.

Venous thrombosis

There is an increased risk of deep venous thrombosis in Behçet's disease, as well as superficial thrombophlebitis.

MANAGEMENT

The drug therapy of Behçet's disease consists of two major elements: first the management of acute exacerbations, and second the prevention of disease relapse. Most patients will require treatment for many years and the potential for iatrogenic complications from therapy is considerable; for these reasons it is important to ensure that therapy is directed at remediable disease.

Management of acute disease

Isolated acute anterior uveitis that is non-sight threatening and with or without hypopyon can be treated with intensive topical steroids and mydriatics/cycloplegics. Colchicine is commonly used for this pattern of disease relapse in Japan, but is not popular in

Western countries and its effectiveness as an ocular therapy has been questioned.[22]

Sight threatening posterior segment disease almost invariably requires systemic therapy with corticosteroids because periocular steroid injections do not allow sufficiently rapid control of disease activity. Prednisolone in a dose of 1–2 mg/kg per day (or equivalent doses of dexamethasone, or methylprednisolone) is administered by mouth in single or divided doses. In Japan, systemic steroids have, in the past, been considered to be ineffective or even detrimental in the treatment of Behçet's disease, and colchicine, which was the drug of first choice there for systemic therapy, has more recently been replaced by cyclosporin A[23-25] or tacrolimus (FK506).[26]

In severe cases, for example, involvement of an only eye or bilateral disease, second line therapy may be initiated early and cyclosporin is the drug of choice in this situation, in a dose of 5 mg/kg per day in two divided doses. Higher dosage regimens of cyclosporin A are inevitably associated with nephrotoxicity, although a dose of 7.5 mg/kg per day may be sufficiently well tolerated for several weeks to allow disease control to be achieved in selected cases. Intravenous pulses of methylprednisolone (500–1000 mg) may also be used to help induce control of intraocular inflammation. Tacrolimus has been used in Japan in a similar way to cyclosporin A with equivalent clinical results, but with the same profile of side effects and less predictable clinical response; it does not appear to offer significant advantage over cyclosporin A.

Long term therapy

The long term visual prognosis in Behçet's disease is poor when assessed over a period of five years or longer.[4, 5] No randomised, controlled, prospective clinical trials of therapy have been undertaken for this length of time in Behçet's disease, and reliable evidence that any particular combination of immunosuppressive or immunomodulatory therapy is particularly effective over this time is lacking. Retrospective studies do, however, suggest that modern immunosuppressive regimens are of benefit in reducing visual morbidity, with one recent series of 28 patients followed for an average of six years reporting retention of an acuity of 6/9 or more in the better eye in 60% of patients.[25] It is important to remember that the cumulative toxicity of drug therapy over this time scale can be considerable, so that appropriate patient counselling and prophylaxis, for example, against steroid induced osteoporosis, must be provided where necessary.

In a two-year, randomised, placebo controlled trial, azathioprine[26] therapy (2.5 mg/kg per day) was shown to reduce the incidence of ophthalmic manifestations of Behçet's disease in Turkish men in two groups: those who had not previously experienced eye problems or in the unaffected fellow eye of those who had disease in one eye. Cyclosporin A therapy has been shown to be superior to monthly cyclophosphamide given by intravenous bolus over a two year period, when it was associated with an initial visual improvement during the first six months, although this improvement was not subsequently sustained.

It has been suggested that chlorambucil treatment may result in induction of a long term clinical remission of disease activity in Behçet's disease,[29, 30] and this hypothesis is worthy of further study. Infertility is a major complication of chlorambucil treatment, however, and although this problem may be minimised by techniques such as sperm banking, chlorambucil's popularity has waned in favour of combination therapy with steroids and cyclosporin A.[31] Cyclosporin A monotherapy is effective in Behçet's disease but associated with greater renal toxicity than combination treatment with steroids.[24, 32]

When ocular inflammation is quiescent, it may not be possible to determine whether this is as a result of drug therapy or natural remission of the disease. In these circumstances, a cautious withdrawal of therapy should be considered after a reasonable period of stability (3–6 months) with reintroduction of therapy as and when necessary.

1 Behçet H. Über rezidivierende Aphthose, durch ein Virus verursachte Geschwüre am Mund, am Auge und an den Genitalien. *Dermatol Wochenschr* 1937;**36**:1152–7.
2 Feigenbaum A. Description of Behçet's syndrome in the Hippocratic third book of endemic diseases. *Br J Ophthalmol* 1956;**40**:355–7.
3 Palimeris G, Koliopoulos G, Theodossiadis G, et al. The Adamantiadis–Behçet's syndrome. *Trans Ophthalmol Soc UK* 1980;**100**:527–30.
4 Mamo JG: The rate of visual loss in Behçet's disease, *Arch Ophthalmol* 1970;**84**:451–2.
5 Benezra D, Cohen E. Treatment and visual prognosis in Behçet's disease. *Br J Ophthalmol* 1986;**70**:589–92.

6 International Study Group for Behçet's disease. Criteria for diagnosis of Behçet's disease. *Lancet* 1990;**335**:1078–80.

7 Behçet's Disease Research Committee of Japan, Health and Welfare of Japan. *Annual Report* 1978:16–17.

8 Colvard DM, Robertson DM, O'Duffy JD. The ocular manifestations of Behçet's disease, *Arch Ophthalmol* 1977;**95**:1813–17.

9 Ohno S, Aoki K, Sugiura S, Itakura K, Aizawa M. HL-A5 and Behçet's disease. *Lancet* 1973;**ii**:1383–4.

10 Ohno S, Ohguchi M, S, Matsuda H, Wakisaka A, Aizawa M. Close association of HLA-Bw51 with Behçet's disease. *Arch Ophthalmol* 1982;**100**:1455–8.

11 Kilmartin DJ, Finch, Acheson RW. Primary association of HLA-B51 with Behçet's disease in Ireland. *Br J Ophthalmol* 1997;**81**:649–53.

12 Mizuki N, Inoko H, Sugimura K, et al. RFLP analysis in the TNF-β gene and the susceptibility to alloreactive NK cells in Behçet's disease. *Invest Ophthalmol Vis Sci* 1992;**33**:3084–90.

13 Feltkamp TEW. Ophthalmological significance of HLA associated uveitis, *Eye* 1990;**4**:839–44

14 Niwa Y, Mizushima Y. Neutrophil-potentiating factors released from stimulated lymphocytes; special reference to the increase in neutrophil-potentiating factors from streptococcus-stimulated lymphocytes of patients with Behçet's disease. *Clin Exp Immunol* 1990;**79**:353–60.

15 Mizushima Y, Matsumura N, Mori M, Shimizu T, Fukushima B, Mimura Y, Saito K, Sugiura S: Colchicine in Behçet's disease. *Lancet* 1977;**ii**:1037.

16 Charteris DG, Champ C, Rosenthal AR, Lightman SL. Behçet's disease: Activated T lymphocytes in retinal perivasculitis. *Br J Ophthalmol* 1992;**76**:499–501.

17 Dinning WJ, Perkins ES. Immunosuppressives in uveitis: a preliminary report of experience with chlorambucil. *Br J Ophthalmol* 1975;**59**:397–403.

18 Bentley CR, Stanford MR, Shilling JS, Sanders MD, Graham EM. Macular ischaemia in posterior uveitis. *Eye* 1993;**7**:411–14.

19 Kalbian VV, Challis MT. Behçet's disease: report of twelve cases with three manifesting as papilledema. *Am J Med* 1970;**49**:823–9.

20 Main DM, Chamberlain MA. Clinical differentiation of oral ulceration in Behçet's disease. *Br J Rheumatol* 1992;**31**:767–70.

21 Jenkins JS, Powell RJ, Allen BR, Littlewood SM, Maurice PD, Smith NJ. Thalidomide in severe orogenital ulceration. *Lancet* 1984;**ii**:1424–6.

22 Aktulga E, Altac M, Muftuoglu A, et al. A double blind study of colchicine in Behçet's disease. *Haematologica* 1980;**65**:399–402.

23 Nussenblatt RB, Palestine AG, Chan CC, Mochizuki M, Yancey K. Effectiveness of cyclosporin therapy for Behçet's disease. *Arthritis Rheum* 1985;**28**:671–9.

24 Masuda K, Nakajima A, Urayama A, et al. Double-masked trial of cyclosporin versus colchicine and long-term open study of cyclosporin in Behçet's disease. *Lancet* 1989;**i**:1093–6.

25 Towler HMA, Lightman S. Visual prognosis in Behçet's disease. *Ocular Immunol Inflam* 1993;**1**:249–54.

26 Mochizuki M, Masuda K, Sokane T, et al. A multicenter open trial of FK 506 in refractory uveitis, including Behçet's disease. Japanese FK 506 study group on refractory uveitis. *Transplant Proc* 1991;**23**:3343–6.

27 Yazici H, Pazarli H, Barnes CG, et al. A controlled trial of azathioprine in Behçet's syndrome. *N Engl J Med* 1990;**322**:281–5.

28 Ozyazgan Y, Yurdakul S, Yazici H, et al. Low dose cyclosporin A versus pulsed cyclophosphamide in Behçet's syndrome: A single masked trial. *Br J Ophthalmol* 1992;**76**:241–3.

29 Abdalla, MI, Baghat, NED. Long-lasting remission of Behçet's disease after chlorambucil therapy, *Br J Ophthalmol* 1973;**57**:706–11.

30 Tessler HH, Jennings T. High-dose short-term chlorambucil for intractable sympathetic ophthalmia and Behçet's disease. *Br J Ophthalmol* 1990;74:353–7.

31 Tabbara KF. Chlorambucil in Behçet's disease: a reappraisal. *Ophthalmology* 1983;90:906–8.

32 Whitcup SM, Salvo EC, Nussenblatt RB. Combined cyclosporine and corticosteroid therapy for sight-threatening uveitis in Behçet's disease. *Am J Ophthalmol* 1994;118:39–45

7: Other disorders affecting the choroid and retina

Involvement of the choroid and retina is common in many forms of ocular inflammation. This inflammation may be diffuse, multifocal, or focal and associated with varying degrees of overlying vitreous inflammation. Each type encompasses a group of disorders which are individually diagnosed largely on their clinical appearances. The inflammation may be located at the level of the neuroretina, the retinal pigment epithelium, the choroid, or more commonly throughout more than one layer. Clinically, it is important to determine the anatomical level of the inflammation because this will help in the differential diagnosis. Treatment for the inflammatory process is as for other forms of ocular inflammation (see chapter 8) or is directed at the infecting organism when relevant (toxoplasmosis and toxocariasis are covered in chapter 5).

DIFFUSE CHORIORETINITIS
Vogt–Koyanagi–Harada syndrome

Vogt–Koyanagi–Harada (VKH) syndrome is a severe bilateral uveitis associated with exudative retinal detachment and signs and symptoms of meningitis. The American Uveitis Society has adopted the following diagnostic criteria: bilateral panuveitis with serous retinal detachment, central nervous system (CNS) manifestations (meningismus, headache, cerebrospinal fluid [CSF] pleocytosis), auditory manifestations (hearing loss, tinnitus), cutaneous manifestations (vitiligo, alopecia, poliosis), and no history of ocular surgery or trauma.

100

VKH syndrome is more common in Asians, Hispanic people, Japanese, American Indians, and Asian Indians. It usually has a rapid onset with headaches and other neurological symptoms, soon followed by uveitis with widespread or multiple serous retinal detachments and optic disc swelling, (Fig 7.1). Fluorescein angiography reveals abnormal choroidal filling and numerous punctate hyperfluorescent dots at the level of the retinal pigment epithelium (RPE), with eventual pooling of the dye. Disc staining is also common. B scan ultrasonography reveals moderate choroidal thickening. Examination of the CSF reveals a sterile

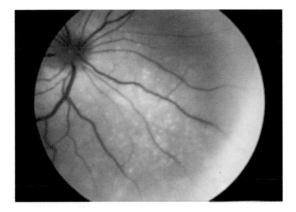

(a)

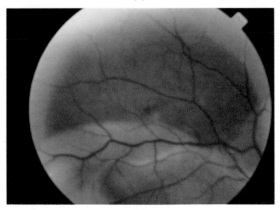

(b)

Figure 7.1   (a) Characteristic pink optic disc and small pale chorioretinal lesions and (b) serous retinal detachment in Vogt–Koyanagi–Harada syndrome.

lymphocytic meningitis. The cutaneous manifestations usually occur in the convalescent phase or well after the active uveitis has resolved. VKH syndrome is associated with the HLA-DR4 antigen and in particular the HLA-DRB1*0405 genotype.

There is usually a prompt response to high doses of oral corticosteroids with resolution characterised by widespread RPE changes. Recurrence (especially chronic anterior uveitis) and the need for long term immunosuppression are not uncommon. The dysacusis usually resolves over several months.

With aggressive systemic immunosuppression, the long term prognosis has improved markedly in VKH syndrome including the group who develop chronic disease.[1] Long term visual loss may arise from chronic macular changes, subretinal neovascularisation, optic nerve damage, cataract formation, or late glaucoma.

Serpiginous choroidopathy

Serpiginous choroidopathy (geographical choroidopathy, geographical helicoid peripapillary choroidopathy) is a rare choroidal inflammatory disorder that is mainly, chronic, progressive, and bilateral, affecting the posterior pole (Fig 7.2). It usually presents in the fourth to fifth decade although it may occur earlier. The symptoms of paracentral scotomata and metamorphopsia are variable and depend on the position of the lesions. Initially the

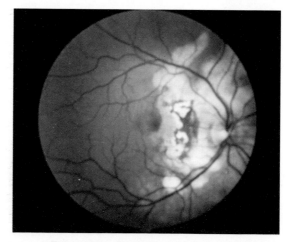

Figure 7.2   Serpiginous choroiditis.

active lesions may appear as isolated areas of choroidal pallor with overlying retinal oedema, progressing over several weeks to months and then resolving to leave well defined areas of chorioretinal atrophy with hyperpigmented borders. Most lesions, however, appear as areas of active inflammation adjacent to previous scars. There is minimal if any overlying vitritis or anterior chamber inflammation. The visual outcome depends on the site of retinal involvement and there is usually little central visual recovery if the macula is involved. The disease progresses in a slow stepwise manner and prolonged remissions are not uncommon. The disease may be complicated by retinal vascular occlusions or subretinal neovascularisation.[2]

Fluorescein angiography of the active lesions shows early hypofluorescence with late staining and may show secondary subretinal neovascularisation. Vision threatening active lesions can be treated with systemic corticosteroids and laser photocoagulation is used to treat subretinal neovascularisation if the lesions are extrafoveal.

Uveal effusion syndrome

This rare condition is characterised by peripheral serous detachment of the choroid occurring in the absence of nanophthalmos, hypotony, scleral inflammation, or recent surgery.[3] The patients may present with peripheral field loss or with central visual loss when the macula becomes involved. It is usually bilateral and there is often an associated overlying serous retinal detachment. B scan ultrasonography reveals the choroidal thickening and peripheral choroidal and ciliary body detachment. In some cases there is ultrasonographic evidence of scleral thickening. Secondary RPE hypertrophy is seen before and after retinal reattachment.

The choroidal effusion is probably caused by poor transscleral fluid flow. This is caused by an accumulation of glycosaminoglycans (dermatan sulphate and chondroitin sulphate) and an increase in collagen fibril width.[4] If persistent the effusions can be treated by partial thickness sclerectomy[5] with or without formal sclerostomy.

Subretinal fibrosis and uveitis syndrome

This is an uncommon condition occurring mainly in women in the third to fifth decades of life. It is usually bilateral and characterised by an acute phase with multifocal choroiditis, usually with minimal signs of anterior chamber or vitreous inflammation. The multifocal chorioretinal lesions are small (100–200 μm), pale, and scattered throughout the posterior pole. Fluorescein angiography may show a lacy network of hyperfluorescence under the active lesions, with late leak less than might be expected from typical subretinal neovascularisation. Serous retinal detachment may occur at the macula with exudate, haemorrhage, and rapid progression to a focal fibrous scar. The lesions gradually scar and coalesce forming broad bands of subretinal fibrosis.[6] The margins of the lesions become pigmented and surrounded by a rim of depigmentation. The final visual outcome is poor with vision usually at the level of 6/60 or worse in affected eyes.

The patients have no apparent associated systemic disease and no treatment is useful after subretinal fibrosis has occurred, although systemic corticosteroids may be useful in treating acute macular lesions.

MULTIFOCAL CHORIO-RETINITIS

Sympathetic ophthalmia

Sympathetic ophthalmia is a well defined entity of bilateral chronic panuveitis with choroidal thickening and inflammation after penetrating injury or surgery[7] (see chapter 4).

Presumed ocular histoplasmosis syndrome

Presumed ocular histoplasmosis syndrome (POHS) is characterised by a clinical triad of peripapillary pigmentary atrophy, subretinal neovascularisation at the macula, and multiple small peripheral atrophic lesions. It is associated with no anterior chamber or vitreous inflammation. The usual age of onset is the fifth decade. Patients generally have no symptoms until there is macular involvement, by which time the peripheral lesions are quiescent. The peripheral lesions are small (200–500 μm), clearly defined (punched out), and depigmented (Fig 7.3). The subretinal neovascularisation usually occurs in association with a visible scar.

Recurrence usually takes the form of new episodes of subretinal neovascularisation.[8]

There is circumstantial epidemiological evidence linking POHS to infection with *Histoplasma capsulatum* in that the ocular disease is much more common in those areas endemic for *Histoplasma capsulatum,* and patients have a high incidence of positive histoplasmin skin tests. It is well established, however, that an identical disease can occur without any evidence of previous exposure to *Histoplasma capsulatum.* Fluorescein angiography shows the subretinal neovascularisation when present; the peripheral atrophic

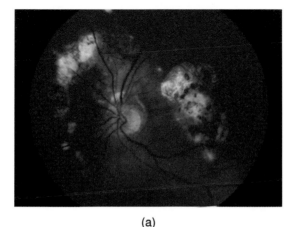

(a)

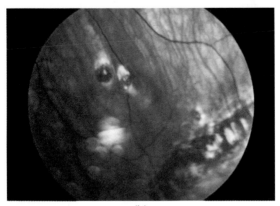

(b)

Figure 7.3   Presumed ocular histoplasmosis syndrome - appearance of chorioretinal lesions at the posterior pole (a) and in the retinal periphery (b).

lesions hyperfluoresce early and then fade with time in the manner of an RPE window defect.

Patients should be warned of the risk of subretinal neovascularisation and its symptoms, and given an Amsler chart to use. Treatment is aimed at photocoagulation of extrafoveal subretinal neovascularisation and is effective at maintaining good central vision unless there is subfoveal involvement, when submacular surgery may be indicated (see chapter 9).

Multifocal choroiditis and panuveitis

Multifocal choroiditis and panuveitis (MCP) is a heterogeneous disorder affecting patients of all ages. It usually has an acute onset and is characterised by prominent anterior chamber and vitreous inflammation. There are multifocal chorioretinal lesions of varying ages and sizes (between 50 and 350 μm). The acute lesions are pale yellow or grey and develop prominent hyperpigmentation as they mature. There is a high incidence of secondary subretinal neovascularisation and macular oedema[9] (Fig 7.4). The site of the lesions is variable and may be in the periphery or posterior pole or both. The disease usually has a relapsing–remitting course and final visual acuity is generally good, unless the macula is directly affected.

Systemic investigation is normal although the disease can be closely mimicked by sarcoidosis and this should be excluded in all cases (see chapter 3). Fluorescein angiography of active lesions

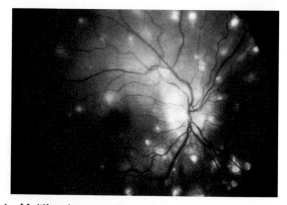

Figure 7.4 Multifocal panuveitis and uveitis with secondary subretinal neovascularisation.

shows early blocking and late staining; older lesions show early hyperfluorescence and late staining typical of window defects of the RPE.

Patients with MCP and visual loss from macular oedema may respond to treatment with systemic corticosteroids but the results of photocoagulation or steroid treatment of subretinal neovascularisation appear poor.

Punctate inner choroidopathy

Punctate inner choroidopathy (PIC) is characterised by an acute onset of multifocal small (100–300 μm) grey or yellow spots scattered around the posterior pole. The lesions are usually bilateral and appear to lie at the level of the RPE or inner choroid. There is minimal if any overlying vitreous inflammation. There may be an overlying sensory retinal detachment. The disease was originally described in young, moderately myopic women who present with blurred vision, scotomata, or photopsia. Usually the degree of visual loss is consistent with the structural damage, but as is seen in multiple evanescent white dot syndrome (MEWDS) there may be field loss unaccounted for by the degree of visible retinal pathology.

The lesions usually resolve forming atrophic retinal scars with or without pigment epithelial proliferation and recurrence is uncommon; there is, however, a high incidence of subretinal neovascularisation.

Fluorescein angiography of the acute lesions shows early hyperfluorescence and late staining. All systemic investigations are usually normal. Treatment is usually restricted to management of subretinal neovascularisation.[10]

Acute posterior multifocal placoid pigment epitheliopathy

Acute posterior multifocal placoid pigment epitheliopathy (APMPPE) presents with acute visual blurring, distortion, or scotomata. It is usually bilateral and affects young adults. Typically APMPPE presents with discrete, plaque like, cream coloured, deep retinal lesions (500–2500 μm in size) with indistinct margins (Fig 7.5). There is mild overlying vitritis in 50% of cases. The lesions are most common in the posterior pole and never occur anterior to the

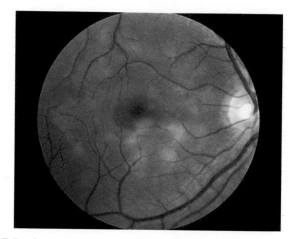

Figure 7.5   Acute posterior multifocal placoid pigment epitheliopathy.

equator. As the lesions mature they lose their creaminess and develop varying degrees of retinal pigmentary mottling, lesions of varying age often coexist. About one third of patients with APMPPE will give a history of a preceding "viral" illness, and a small minority of patients will have evidence of coexisting systemic or cerebral vasculitis.[11]

Fluorescein angiography of the lesions shows absence of the early choroidal fluorescence followed by late staining. Inactive lesions appear as RPE transmission defects without late hyperfluorescence. Indocyanine green angiography demonstrates choroidal flow abnormalities under the placoid lesions, suggesting choroidal hypoperfusion or choroidal vascular inflammation as the cause of APMPPE.[12]

Most often the disease occurs in an acute self limiting form and resolves without treatment over a period of weeks, leaving relative scotomata relating to the site of the placoid lesions. Large submacular lesions will result in poor vision. When recurrent disease occurs, it usually does so within 6 months. Even with recurrent disease, there is little evidence of effectiveness of treatment and, as with all focal outer retinal lesions, subretinal neovascularisation may occur.

Birdshot choroidoretinopathy

In 1980 Ryan and Maumenee[13] described a syndrome characterised by multiple, small (less than a quarter disc diameter), oval,

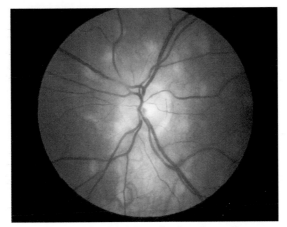

Figure 7.6   Birdshot chorioretinopathy.

cream coloured, outer retinal or choroidal lesions with ill defined margins scattered around the optic disc, nasal fundus, and midperiphery and radiating towards the equator (Fig 7.6). The disease has a gradual onset, presenting with floaters and followed by gradual central visual loss. It has a predilection for women aged between 40 and 70 years. Other typical clinical features are minimal anterior segment inflammation with mild to moderate vitritis, depigmentation of the lesions without pigment migration or hyperpigmentation, narrowing of the retinal arterioles with vasculitis, and occasional flame shaped haemorrhages. Macular oedema and disc oedema are both common.

Fluorescein angiography may show little or no abnormality in the region of the birdshot lesions. Prominent disc and macular oedema may be evident in the later stages. Systemic associations are uncommon but 95% of patients carry the HLA-A29 antigen[14] which can be used to confirm the diagnosis.

The usual course is chronic and, progressive and, as with other multifocal outer retinal lesions, subretinal new vessels may form. The long term visual outcome is limited by chronic macular changes. Effective treatment requires long term moderate immunosuppression.

Multiple evanescent white dot syndrome

In 1984 Jampol described a syndrome of small (100–200 μm) discrete white spots at the level of the RPE located mainly at the posterior pole. The syndrome is usually (but not always) unilateral, acute, and occurs in young (second and third decade), otherwise healthy women.[15] The patients present with visual loss, scotomata, and photopsia. There may be visual field loss in excess of that predicted from the fundoscopic signs. Other typical clinical features are mild disc swelling, enlargement of the blind spot, and minimal (if any) overlying vitritis. There is generally fine granularity of the fovea after resolution.

Fluorescein angiography shows early granular pinpoint hyperfluorescence of the lesions with late staining, and the electroretinogram (ERG) may show a reduced amplitude suggestive of widespread outer retinal (photoreceptor) dysfunction. The prognosis untreated is good and recurrence is unusual but can occur.[16] In some patients with MEWDS there is a tendency to subretinal neovascularisation.

Acute retinal pigment epitheliitis

Acute retinal pigment epitheliitis (Krill's disease) is an uncommon disease characterised by acute unilateral or bilateral mild central visual blurring or metamorphopsia. The typical lesion is a deep, and grey, outer retinal (RPE) lesion with a yellow rim although the entire lesion may be pale. The lesions occur in clusters of one to four at the posterior pole and may have a honeycomb pattern. There is usually no overlying vitritis although some may occur. Fluorescein angiography of the acute lesions reveals progressive staining of the affected RPE.[17] The lesions are thought to be caused by an acute viral RPE infection[18] untreated the prognosis is good and almost complete visual recovery is the rule.

FOCAL CHORIORETINAL INFLAMMATION

Unilateral acute idiopathic maculopathy

Unilateral acute idiopathic maculopathy was described by Yanuzzi in 1991.[19] It occurs in young adults who present with an acute severe unilateral visual loss, usually after a viral illness. The visual loss is the result of an exudative maculopathy with a serous retinal detachment overlying an area of RPE thickening and pallor.

There is usually a minimal to mild overlying vitritis. The fluorescein angiogram shows early hypofluorescence, presumably resulting from blockage at the level of the RPE, and late hyperfluorescence of the entire lesion. There may be an associated papillitis and bilateral disease is rare.[20] Untreated the prognosis is good and visual recovery to near normal with residual pigmentary change is the norm, unless subretinal choroidal neovascularisation occurs.

DIFFERENTIAL DIAGNOSIS
Choroiditis secondary to systemic inflammatory disease

In all patients with diffuse, multifocal, or unifocal choroidal disease, an underlying systemic disease should be suspected. Sarcoidosis (see chapter 3) can cause a variety of clinical pictures with choroidal involvement, but the most typical ones are panuveitis with multifocal choroiditis with or without retinal vasculitis. Systemic lupus erythematosus can cause choroidal disease through immune complex mediated choroidal vasculitis, leading to multiple serous retinal and RPE detachments. This usually occurs in association with retinal microvascular changes with minimal or no vitritis. Behçet's disease can cause widespread multifocal retinal lesions with vasculitis and prominent uveitis (see chapter 6).

Intra-ocular lymphoma

Intraocular lymphoma can present with a wide range of clinical features. The diagnosis should be considered in any elderly patient with chronic vitritis with or without multifocal chorioretinal lesions. The diagnosis may be made by demonstration of lymphoma in the CNS or elsewhere (by Computed Tomography or MRI or by finding lymphomatous cells in the CSF) or on vitreous biopsy (see chapter 2).

Infectious chorioretinitis

Many primary intraocular infections or metastatic intraocular infections can cause a choroiditis or retinitis and mimic chorio-

111

Table 7.1 Infective causes of retinitis and chorioretinitis

Focal retinitis or chorioretinitis	Multifocal retinitis or chorioretinitis	Diffuse retinitis or chorioretinitis
Toxoplasma gondii	Pneumocystis carinii	Cytomegalovirus
Toxocara canis	Cryptococcus neoformans	Herpes simplex virus
Other nematodes (diffuse subacute neuroretinitis)	Mycobacterium (tuberculosis or atypical)	Varicella-zoster virus
Brucella abortus	Treponema pallidum	Measles virus (SSPE)
Candida spp.	Toxoplasma gondii	Rubella virus (congenital)
Aspergillus fumigatus	Histoplasma spp.	Treponema pallidum
Mycobacterium spp. (tuberculosis or atypical)	Epstein–Barr virus	Onchocerca volvulus
Treponema pallidum	HTLV-1	Borrelia burgdorferi
Bartonella hensii		
Other bacterial		

retinal inflammation from non-infectious causes. These may be unifocal, multifocal, or diffuse. Unifocal metastatic chorioretinal infection is seen in both the immunocompetent and the immuno-compromised host, but multifocal metastatic chorioretinal infection is much more commonly seen in patients with AIDS.[21] (see Table 7.1).

Cytomegalovirus retinitis

The first clinical description of cytomegalovirus (CMV) retinitis was made in 1971.[22] The patient was a 32 year old woman who was a renal transplant recipient and who died and had widespread systemic CMV disease. Before the AIDS pandemic, CMV retinitis was rare and the treatment of CMV retinitis was poor. In 1983, Holland and others made the initial report of the common ocular manifestations of AIDS.[23] The findings included cotton wool spots, retinal haemorrhages (HIV retinopathy), and CMV retinitis.

Cytomegalovirus retinitis is a disease of the severely immunodeficient and in AIDS patients it almost never occurred with a CD4 count of greater than 50 cells/μl.[24] This situation is now different given the advent of highly active anti-retroviral therapy (HAART), with which the CD4 + count may rise although the effect of this on specific immunity to CMV is currently unknown.[25] Cytomegalovirus serology is of little use in the diagnosis of retinitis in AIDS patients, because of the high background level of seropositivity among sexually active gay men and the lack of a rise in titre of

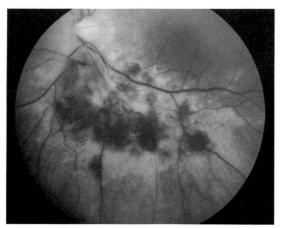

Figure 7.7   Cytomegalovirus retinitis in a patient with AIDS.

CMV antibody during the development of CMV retinitis.[26] Cytomegalovirus serology may occasionally be useful in diagnosing retinitis in non-homosexual AIDS patients, because these patients have a lower background incidence of positive CMV serology.[27]

Cytomegalovirus retinitis appears as confluent areas of full thickness necrotising retinitis with haemorrhage (Fig 7.7). It is often associated with an accompanying retinal vasculitis (which may be severe) and overlying vitritis, which is usually minimal but may be significant if the CD4 count is higher or the patient is on HAART therapy.[25] There may be initial involvement at the posterior pole or in the periphery; when the disease occurs in the periphery it has a more granular appearance than when it occurs at the posterior pole. Occasionally patients with small focal areas of involvement present a diagnostic problem. Visual loss in CMV retinitis may arise from optic nerve or macular involvement with retinitis, rhegmatogenous retinal detachment, serous macular detachment, or cystoid macular oedema. Of these causes only serous or rhegmatogenous detachment is reversible.

Treatment of the CMV retinitis is with drugs, all of which are currently virostatic, and drugs to improve the patients' immune status and decrease the circulating HIV viral load. The antiviral drugs include ganciclovir, foscarnet, and cidofovir, and treatment may be given either locally into the eye (with ganciclovir or foscarnet, either by intravitreal injection or implant [ganciclovir only at present]) or systemically either intravenously (ganciclovir, foscarnet, and cidofovir)[28] or orally (ganciclovir). The principles of treatment are to induce remission with induction treatment and then to maintain remission with secondary prophylaxis while monitoring for relapse.[29] In addition, consideration is also now given to improving the immune function by decreasing the viral load with HAART therapy.

After treatment, the clinical appearance of the retinitis changes; healed retinitis is easily recognised by a lack of retinal thickening (seen as a loss of retinal whitening) with disappearance of retinal haemorrhage and vasculitis, and halting of progression of the retinitis. Occasionally there is an atypical healing response with persistence of a white flat border of opacification[30] which does not advance for many weeks to months. The incidence of bilateral disease and retinal detachment increases with increasing survival of patients with CMV retinitis and extensive peripheral disease.[31] Detachment occurs as a result of a combination of multiple small peripheral retinal holes, posterior vitreous detachment, and a mild degree of proliferative vitreoretinopathy.

Acute retinal necrosis

Acute retinal necrosis (ARN or BARN [bilateral]) is a rapidly progressive viral retinitis. It was first described in 1971[32] and the clinical features have been summarised by the American Uveitis Society.[33] Its suggested criteria for the use of the term may be summarised as: one or more foci of retinal necrosis with discrete borders primarily located in the peripheral retina (Fig 7.8), rapid circumferential progression of the disease (if untreated), occlusive

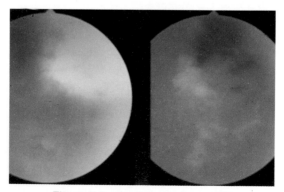

Figure 7.8   Acute retinal necrosis.

vasculopathy with arteriolar involvement, and a prominent inflammatory reaction in the vitreous and anterior chamber. Characteristics that support, but are not required for, the diagnosis include: optic neuritis/atrophy, scleritis, pain, and early retinal detachment.

Initially ARN was described in immunocompetent patients but, recently, a very similar clinical variant has been seen in patients with AIDS.[34] When it occurs in AIDS patients it is frequently preceded by cutaneous herpes zoster infection. Acute retinal necrosis may occasionally follow a mild self limiting course.[35]

The usual causative organism is varicella-zoster virus but herpes simplex types I and II and CMV have all been implicated.[36, 37] The causative organism may be identified, when there is a diagnostic dilemma, by vitreous or retinal microscopy or culture, evidence of intraocular antibody production, or polymerase chain reaction techniques.

Treatment is with high dose antiviral therapy and intravenous acyclovir/famciclovir[38] is used, which may decrease the early incidence of BARN,[39] and laser treatment around the affected areas as prophylaxis against retinal detachment occurring in the future. The visual outlook is generally poor and visual loss, when it occurs, is the result of macular involvement with retinitis, optic papillitis (and subsequent atrophy), or retinal detachment, which often requires vitrectomy with silicone tempiuaele. Second eye involvement may occur many years later.

Progressive outer retinal necrosis

Progressive outer retinal necrosis (PORN) is a recently described clinical variant of necrotising herpetic retinopathy in patients with AIDS.[40] It is caused by varicella-zoster virus infection of the retina. Its course and clinical features distinguish it from ARN and CMV retinopathy. Early on the disease is characterised by multifocal deep retinal opacification at the posterior pole (Fig 7.9). The lesions rapidly coalesce and progress to total retinal necrosis over a short period of time. Despite aggressive therapy with intravenous antiviral drugs, the prognosis is poor; disease progression and/or recurrence is common and most patients develop no light perception vision. The most effective therapy to date involves combinations of antiviral drugs. Total retinal detachments are common. Prophylaxis against retinal detachment using laser

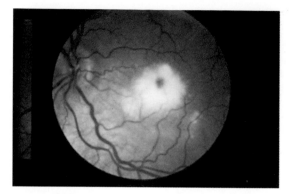

Figure 7.9   Progressive outer retinal necrosis in a patient with AIDS.

retinopexy has not been useful in most cases. PORN is an uncommon, but devastating, complication of AIDS.

1   Moorthy RS, Inomata H, Rao NA. Vogt–Koyanagi–Harada syndrome. *Surv Ophthalmol* 1995;39:265–92.
2   El–Asrar AMA. Serpiginous (geographical) choroiditis. *Int Ophthalmol Clin* 1995; 35:87–91.
3   Stelmach MZ, O'Day J, Ryan H. Uveal effusion syndrome. *Aust NZ J Ophthalmol.* 1994;22:139–43.
4   Forrester JV, Lee WR, Kerr PR, Dua HS. The uveal effusion syndrome and trans-scleral flow. *Eye* 1990;4:354–65.
5   Johnson MW, Gass JDM. Surgical management of the idiopathic uveal effusion syndrome. *Ophthalmology* 1990;97:778–85.
6   Cantrill HL, Folk JC. Multifocal choroiditis associated with progressive subretinal fibrosis. *Am J Ophthalmol* 1986;101:170–80.
7   Chan C C. Relationship between sympathetic ophthalmia, phacoanaphylactic endophthalmitis, and Vogt–Koyanagi–Harada disease. *Ophthalmology* 1988;95:619–23.
8   Tiedeman JS. An approach to the patient with multifocal chorioretinal disease: presumed ocular histoplasmosis syndrome and its fundascopic mimics. *Semin Ophthalmol* 1991;6:2–20.
9   Dreyer RF, Gass JDM. Multifocal choroiditis and panuveitis — a syndrome that mimics ocular histoplasmosis. *Arch Ophthalmol* 1984;102:1776–84.
10 Watzke RC, Packer AJ, Folk JC, Benson WE, Burgess D, Ober RR. Punctate inner choroidopathy. Am J Ophthalmol 1984; 98:572–84.
11 Jones NP. Acute posterior multifocal pigment epitheliopathy. *Br J Ophthalmol* 1995;79:384–9.
12 Yuzawa M, Kawamura A, Matsui M. Indocyanine green video angiographic findings in acute posterior multifocal placoid pigment epitheliopathy. *Acta Ophthalmol* 1994;72:128–33.
13 Ryan SJ, Maumenee AE. Birdshot retinochoroidopathy. *Am J Ophthalmol* 1980;89:31–45.
14 Priem HA, Oosterhuis JA. Birdshot chorioretinopathy: clinical characteristics and evolution. *Br J Ophthalmol* 1988; 72:646–59.
15 Reddy CV, Brown J Jr, Folk JC, Kimura AE, Gupta S, Walker J, Jampol LM.Enlarged blind spots in chorioretinal inflammatory disorders. *Ophthalmology* 1996;103:606–17.

16 Tsai L, Jampol LM, Pollock SC, Olk J. Chronic recurrent multiple evanescent white dot syndrome *Retina* 1994;14:160–3.
17 Luttrull JK. Acute retinal pigment epitheliitis. *Am J Ophthalmol* 1997;123:127–9.
18 Krill AE, Deutman AF. Acute retinal pigment epitheliitis. *Am J Ophthalmol* 1972;74:193–205.
19 Yannuzzi LA, Jampol LM, Rabb MF, Sorenson JA, Beyrer C, Wilcox LM Jr. Unilateral acute idiopathic maculopathy. *Arch Ophthalmol.* 1991;109:1411–16.
20 Freund KB, Yannuzzi LA, Barile GR, Spaide RF, Milewski SA, Guyer DR. The expanding clinical spectrum of unilateral acute idiopathic maculopathy. *Arch Ophthalmol* 1996;114:555–9.
21 Rosenblatt MA, Cunningham C, Teich S, Friedman AH. Choroidal lesions in patients with AIDS. *Br J Ophthalmol* 1990;74:610–14.
22 de Venecia G, Rhein GMZ, Pratt MV, Kisken W. Cytomegalic inclusion retinitis in an adult. *Arch Ophthalmol* 1971;86:44–57.
23 Holland GN, Pepose JS, Pettit TH, Gottlieb MS, Yee RD, Foos RY. Acquired immune deficiency syndrome ocular manifestations. *Ophthalmology* 1983;90:859–72.
24 Crowe SM, Carlin JB, Stewart KI, Lucas CR, Hoy JF. Predictive value of lymphocyte CD4 numbers for the development of opportunistic infections and malignancies in HIV infected persons. *J AIDS* 1991;4:770–6.
25 Jacobson MA, Zegans M, Pavan PR et al. Cytomegalovirus retinitis after initiation of highly active anti-retroviral therapy. *Lancet* 1997;349:1443–5.
26 Lazzarotto T, Dal Monte P, Boccuni MC, Ripalti A, Landini MP. Lack of correlation between virus detection and serologic tests for diagnosis of active cytomegalovirus infection in patients with AIDS. *J Clin Microbiol* 1992;30:1027–9.
27 Jackson JB, Erice A, Englund JA, Edson JR, Balfour HH. Prevalence of cytomegalovirus antibody in haemophiliacs and homosexuals infected with human immunodeficiency virus type 1. *Transfusion* 1988;28:187–9.
28 Lalezari JP, Stagg RJ, Kupperman BD et al. Intravenous cidofovir for peripheral cytomegalovirus retinis in patients with AIDS. A randomised controlled trial. *Ann Intern Med* 1997;126:257–63.
29 Hardy WD. Management strategies for patients with cytomegalovirus retinitis. *J AIDS Hum Retrovirol* 1997;14:S7–12.
30 Keefe KS, Freeman WR, Peterson TJ, Wiley CA, Crapotta J, Quiceno JI, Listhaus AD. Atypical healing of cytomegalovirus retinitis. Significance of persistent border opacification. *Ophthalmology* 1992;99:1377–84.
31 Jabs DA, Enger C, Haller J, de Bustros S. Retinal detachments in patients with cytomegalovirus retinitis. *Arch Ophthalmol* 1991;109:794–9.
32 Urayama A, Yamada N, Sasaki T, et al. Unilateral acute uveitis with retinal periarteritis and detachment. *Jpn J Clin Ophthalmol* 1971;25:607–19.
33 Holland GN and the Executive Committee of the American Uveitis Society. Standard diagnostic criteria for the acute retinal necrosis syndrome. *Am J Ophthalmol* 1994;117:663–7.
34 Batisse D, Eliaszewicz M, Zazoun L, Baudrimont M, Pialoux G, Dupont B. Acute retinal necrosis in the course of AIDS: study of 26 cases. *AIDS* 1996;10:55–60.
35 Matsuo T, Nakayama T, Koyama T, Koyama M, Matsuo N. A proposed mid type of acute retinal necrosis syndrome. *Am J Ophthalmol* 1988;105:579–83.
36 Pepose JS, Flowers B, Stewart JA, Grose C, Levy DS, Culbertson WW, Kreiger AE. Herpesvirus antibody levels in the etiologic diagnosis of the acute retinal necrosis syndrome. *Am J Ophthalmol* 1992;113:248–56.
37 Rahhal FM, Siegel LM, Russak V, et al. Clinicopathologic correlations in acute retinal necrosis caused by herpes simplex virus type 2. *Arch Ophthalmol* 1996;114:1416–9.

38 Figueroa MS, Garabito I, Gutierrez C, Fortun J. Famciclovir for the treatment of acute retinal necrosis (ARN) sysndrome. *Am J Ophthalmol* 1977;**123**:255–7.
39 Palay DA, Sternberg P Jr, Davis J, et al. Decrease in the risk of bilateral acute retinal necrosis by aciclovir therapy. *Am J Ophthalmol.* 1991;**112**:250–5.
40 Holland GN. The progressive outer retinal necrosis syndrome. *Int Ophthalmol* 1994;**18**:163–5.

8: Assessment and medical management of posterior uveitis and its complications

Patients with intraocular inflammatory disease often lose vision or have visual symptoms for a variety of reasons.[1] Thorough clinical examination of the eye is necessary to determine the cause or causes of this, because there may be more than one reason and clinical judgment is vital as to the relative significance of each. Visual loss is not inevitable and many patients may only have mild symptoms, for example, floaters are a common complaint. Each patient must be individually appraised and their visual difficulties determined in detail. Patients' visual needs differ greatly, and what is a mild problem for one may be a severe handicap for another. All intervention, be it medical or surgical, has the potential for complications, and therapy of any sort should be embarked upon only when it is clearly indicated and necessary.

EXAMINATION OF THE EYE

The recording of visual acuity is the start of most ophthalmic assessments and in patients with uveitis can yield a great deal of useful information. For example, the patient with visually significant floaters may attempt to flick them out of the way to facilitate reading the chart letters, or may wait for them to settle before attempting the next line. Patients with macular problems may read with eccentric fixation or complain that the letters are distorted. Ambient lighting may have a significant effect on functional vision. Glare in bright sunlight or dazzle from car headlights may be a major problem for the patient with posterior subcapsular lens opacities, so that good vision under clinic conditions needs to be interpreted with functional information from the patient.

All ocular structures need to be examined so that the full extent of involvement by the inflammatory process and the relative contribution of each element to overall visual dysfunction can be ascertained. For example, band keratopathy, corneal neovascularisation, melting and scars, corneal oedema, and extensive keratic precipitates on the corneal endothelium may all result in visual impairment. Examination of the anterior chamber for cells, flare and fibrin, iris for nodules, posterior and anterior synechiae, transillumination defects, lens for opacities and so on through the eye is carried out. The intraocular pressure is measured, afferent pupillary defects examined for, and the pupils dilated before fundal examination. Very careful examination of the posterior segment is vital to determine if there is vitritis, posterior vitreous detachment, retinitis, choroiditis, retinal vasculitis (arterial or venous), or any abnormality of the optic nerve and macula. Good visualisation of the peripheral retina is very important when examining the eye in uveitis, with particular regard to the detection of pars plana snowbanks, vitreous snowballs, or vitreoretinal abnormalities. Careful assessment of the posterior segment, together with fluorescein angiography and electrodiagnostic tests such as visual evoked response (VER) or electroretinogram (ERG), where appropriate, will allow the cause(s) of visual loss to be determined.

It is important to be constantly aware of diagnostic pitfalls, and consideration should always be given to an underlying infective aetiology (for example, varicella-zoster virus or metastatic endophthalmitis) or intraocular neoplasia (for example, B cell lymphoma) (see chapter 7).

MANAGEMENT PRINCIPLES

Anterior uveitis

When associated with posterior uveitis, anterior uveitis should be assessed and treated using the same criteria as when it occurs in isolation (see chapter 1).

120

Indications for intervention in posterior uveitis

Intraocular inflammatory disease requires treatment when the inflammatory process is threatening the sight or causing damage to the eye.[2] As indicated above, the visual requirements of individual patients can vary considerably and what is a minor problem for one may cause a major problem for another. Unilateral disease may not be a practical problem to the patient with a normal fellow eye, which nevertheless may require treatment for active inflammation.

Management of inflammatory signs in posterior uveitis

Whether ocular inflammation is associated with a systemic disease or not, the management of the inflammatory process (masquerade syndromes having been excluded) depends on the nature and extent of ocular involvement and not the underlying disorder, with the exception of toxoplasma chorioretinitis (see chapter 5). The principles of treatment are the same whatever the clinical disease entity, which is reflected by the fact that the immunopathology of these disorders is very similar.[3] The posterior segment ocular complications most commonly requiring medical treatment are vitritis and macular oedema; others include retinitis, especially when the posterior pole is involved, serous retinal detachment, papillitis, optic neuritis, and retinal neovascularisation (see later). If an adequate view of the macula cannot be obtained, fluorescein angiography or fluoroscopy may be required to determine if oedema is present and help identify the causes of visual loss, before consideration of immunosuppressive therapy.

DRUGS USED TO CONTROL THE INFLAMMATORY PROCESS

Corticosteroids

These drugs are the mainstay in the management of inflammatory eye disease.

Local administration

In unilateral disease or in situations where systemic therapy is preferably avoided, for example, pregnancy, periocular steroids may be helpful.[4] These can be delivered by a variety of routes, for example, as an orbital floor or posterior sub-Tenon's injection of a depot or long acting steroid, such as methylprednisolone (Depomedrone) or triamcinolone (Kenalog). The principal contra-indication to the use of long acting steroid injections is raised intraocular pressure at any time.

Periocular steroids are most useful in controlling vitritis and to a lesser extent macular oedema, and a significant number of patients obtain visual improvement.[4] The maximum effect can take several weeks to occur and the duration of benefit is variable. Repeat injections can be performed if there is recurrence of inflammation, and bilateral injections can also be employed.

Systemic steroids

When periocular steroids are ineffectual or disease is bilateral, systemic steroid therapy is commenced. The dose and duration of treatment depend very much on individual circumstances, the duration of therapy being particularly difficult to predict in the early stages.[2, 5] In mild to moderate inflammation, defined as a moderate reduction in vision of about 6/18 or better in which there is no destructive process, an initial dose of prednisolone 0.5–1 mg/kg per day can be used, which approximates to 40 mg/day for an average man. The dose is then titrated downwards against the visual acuity and inflammatory signs, with the aim of controlling the inflammation on the lowest dose of steroid. Many patients will require a small maintenance dose of steroid of 5–10 mg/day for some time because the underlying inflammatory process is unlikely to remit quickly.

In patients with severe, sight threatening inflammation, high dose steroids are required to achieve rapid control, and a dose of prednisolone 1–2 mg/kg per day is required, that is, about 80 mg/day for the average man. This dose is then tapered as the signs improve and the inflammation is brought under control.

Corticosteroids can also be given as an intravenous pulse, usually 500–1000 mg methylprednisolone, which can be repeated every two or three days according to response. Although some authors have found intravenous pulse steroids to be very effective therapy,[5, 6] caution in their use is required because acute cardiovascular collapse can be precipitated and patients must be carefully selected. A poor response to intravenous steroids does not necessarily predict a poor response to oral therapy, and long term use of intravenous steroids may not be practical.

Corticosteroids can have serious systemic side effects including hypertension, diabetes, and acute psychosis, and in the longer term osteoporosis is a particular problem in older patients which requires careful monitoring including bone densitometry, with appropriate prophylaxis where indicated.

A poor response to steroid therapy may be for any of three reasons: the dose of steroids was inadequate; additional immunosuppressive therapy in combination with steroids is necessary; or the disease has caused irreversible damage to critical visual structures and there is no potential for visual recovery. When this latter situation is encountered, a trial of maximum therapy may be required to assess if there is any potential for visual recovery, and high dose steroids in combination with an additional immunosuppressive agent are used.

Additional immunosuppressive agents

In most situations, it is possible to control intraocular inflammation effectively with corticosteroids alone. When, however, there is an inadequate response to steroids or the inflammation can only be controlled on an unacceptably high maintenance dose of steroids (>0.25 mg/kg per day or $>10-15$ mg/day in adults), the addition of a second agent may be beneficial.

Cyclosporin

The choice of second agent depends on many factors including the age and general health of the patient. In otherwise healthy people under the age of 50 years, cyclosporin A is an effective drug. Treatment is usually started at a dose of 5 mg/kg per day, although lower starting doses have been used.[2, 5, 7-10] Beneficial effects on intraocular inflammation are not usually seen for 2–3 weeks, at which time the steroid dose can be reduced. If no improvement has occurred or the steroid dose cannot be successfully reduced, cyclosporin A should be slowly tapered and stopped. Patients should have regular monitoring of serum creatinine, liver function tests, and full blood count; plasma drug levels are rarely helpful for clinical management, unless non-compliance is suspected or untoward side effects have been experienced.[11, 12] A rise in serum creatinine necessitates reduction in cyclosporin A dose and, should the creatinine remain elevated, then cyclosporin A should be completely withdrawn.

In most patients, the steroid dose can be reduced slowly down to an acceptable maintenance level of about 10 mg, the rate of reduction being determined by clinical response. The average patient requiring combination treatment is likely to need the additional therapy for about one year, but there is considerable variation in response, from a few months to many years, and it is impossible to predict this at the outset of therapy. Dose reduction of both agents should be done slowly, and this is particularly important with cyclosporin A because rebound inflammation can occur.[13]

Azathioprine

In older patients or those who are unable to tolerate cyclosporin A, azathioprine is the drug of choice, with a starting dose of 2 mg/kg per day in three divided doses up to a maximum of 200 mg daily. Beneficial effects are not seen for several weeks which limits azathioprine's usefulness in the acute situation.[2, 5, 14, 15] The differential white cell count should be monitored and the dose of azathioprine adjusted as necessary.

Cytotoxic agents, cyclophosphamide, and chlorambucil

In patients with Wegener's granulomatosis, cyclophosphamide can be particularly useful, as well as in selected cases of other causes of severe intraocular inflammation.[16] Its toxicity, in both the short and longer term, limit its use in this cohort of patients who are often young. Chlorambucil used to be used extensively as a second line agent in Behçet's disease but its toxicity, which is very similar to cyclophosphamide, limits its use and it has been largely superseded by other agents such as cyclosporin A.[17, 18]

OTHER DRUGS THAT MAY HAVE A ROLE

Methotrexate

Methotrexate has been found to be very useful in the management of rheumatoid arthritis in which it is used as a second line agent, after non-steroidal anti-inflammatory drugs.[19] It is given as a once weekly oral pulse dose (12.5 mg/week or less) with few serious side effects and, although its exact mode of action at this low dose remains uncertain, its anti-proliferative effect is thought to be important.[20, 21] There have been a few studies of its use in intraocular inflammation and it would appear to have a role in patients who are resistant to or cannot tolerate other additional agents. The response time ranges from three to nine weeks[22, 23] so its use is restricted to management of chronic intraocular inflammation rather than acute disease. In one series, methotrexate was found to be more effective in treating patients with inflammatory pseudotumour, scleritis, and orbital myositis rather than intraocular inflammation.

In patients given 40 mg methotrexate intravenously once weekly for four weeks followed by 15 mg/week given orally, intraocular inflammation improved and was associated with significant visual improvement in many.[22] In another study, patients with endogenous uveitis resistant to treatment with high doses of cortisone and other immunosuppressive agents were treated with cyclosporin A (at an initial dose of 5 mg/kg per day, and subsequently modified according to individual clinical response), fluocortolone and methotrexate.[24] Disease remission was obtained in all patients, together with significant improvement in visual acuity and no signs of renal or hepatic toxicity were observed in any of the patients.

Tacrolimus (FK506)

Tacrolimus is a very similar drug to cyclosporin A in its mechanism of action and its use in patients has been largely limited to a few centres, particularly in the transplantation field. Most of the published studies of its use in uveitis have come from Japan. In several open, uncontrolled, multicentre clinical trials to evaluate the efficacy and adverse side effects of single therapy with tacrolimus in refractory uveitis,[25–27] some benefit was found. Both the therapeutic effect and side effects were dose dependent, the major side effects being renal impairment, neurological symptoms, gastrointestinal symptoms, and hyperglycaemia. The definition of refractory uveitis may not mean resistant to corticosteroids and other immunosuppresive agents in these studies, because the use of steroids in Japan may be different from those used in Europe and the USA. Tacrolimus is, however, being increasingly used in organ transplantation, with particular emphasis on its efficacy as monotherapy without concomitant use of steroids, and whether it can permit a lower dose of steroids to be used after transplantation (that is, its steroid sparing effect).

NEW APPROACHES UNDER EVALUATION

Anti-CD4+ monoclonal antibodies

It is known that CD4+ T cells are important in the perpetuation of posterior uveitis and anti-CD4+ T cell therapy using monoclonal antibodies has been used in the management of other auto immune diseases known to involve CD4+ cells.[28] A patient with long standing, refractory, endogenous uveitis was treated with a chimaeric monoclonal anti-CD4 antibody given intravenously.[29] No immediate improvement was documented, but the frequency of uveitis relapses was sharply reduced after this therapy. Interestingly, they report that the patient's response to conventional therapy used to treat the relapses also improved after this treatment. Therapy with these chimaeric antibodies is still limited as a result of the host antibody response engendered by them which limits further use.

Induction of immune tolerance as therapy

Experimental studies have shown that feeding or mucosal administration of retinal proteins and peptides can induce a state of immune tolerance so that the animals are protected from disease.[30, 31] In an open pilot study, patients fed large doses of retinal antigens were able to reduce their dose of immunosuppresive drugs or stop them altogether, and remain in remission with good disease control on no therapy.[32] This has also occurred in patients with multiple sclerosis who were fed myelin basic protein.[33] In a randomised masked trial, patients with endogenous uveitis on drug therapy received either retinal S-antigen or a mixture of retinal antigens or placebo by mouth, the aim being to taper immunosuppresive therapy and observe whether disease remission was maintained. The results of the groups treated by placebo or retinal antigen were not statistically significant, although there was a trend for patients receiving retinal S-antigen to be more likely to have their drug therapy tapered and stopped; a full scale clinical trial is planned.[34]

Intraocular drug administration

Steroids are given to patients with uveitis by a variety of routes and intraocular steroid is often used intraoperatively in patients undergoing vitrectomy for endophthalmitis.[35] Dexamethasone, the steroid currently used, has a very short half life in the eye, however, particularly when the blood–ocular barriers are damaged.[36] Many drugs can be administered via the intraocular route (amikacin, vancomycin, amphotericin B, ganciclovir, and foscarnet to name some) but, in chronic conditions, longer term intraocular drug delivery would be more ideal. In the management of cytomegalovirus (CMV) retinitis in AIDS patients, repeated intravitreal injections of ganciclovir are often used very effectively,[37] avoiding the systemic side effects of the drug but allowing good control of the CMV retinal disease. Slow-release devices filled with ganciclovir[38] are now available for insertion into the eye to avoid the necessity of repeated injections, and can be safely exchanged several times when they no longer contain drug.[39] In time, other drugs such as steroids and cyclosporin A will be available in these devices for treatment of chronic inflammatory ocular problems.[40] If patients with localised ocular disease could be effectively managed entirely by locally administered drugs, a significant advance would have been made over systemic administration which, although effective, has been associated with severe side effects, particularly in those patients of all age groups who require prolonged therapy.

MANAGEMENT OF COMPLICATIONS

Raised intraocular pressure

About 20% of patients with uveitis experience elevation of intraocular pressure at some time during the course of disease.[40] This may be associated with either an open or closed angle mechanism, or in response to steroid therapy, most commonly to local steroid treatment (topical or periocular) and less commonly to systemic administration.

In most patients in whom the drainage angle is open, the elevation of pressure is transient, and not associated with visible optic nerve damage or visual field loss. Treatment where indicated depends on the extent of pressure elevation, and topical therapy, for example β-blockers, α_2-agonists, or topical carbonic anhydrase

127

inhibitors such as dorzolamide, may prove adequate, but, if not, systemic carbonic anhydrase inhibitors such as acetazolamide may be necessary.[41] It is important to maintain control of intraocular inflammation, and to assess if there is any element of steroid responsiveness. The intraocular pressure (IOP) may fall to normal levels with control of inflammation, allowing hypotensive medication to be withdrawn, but if it remains elevated, chronic hypotensive therapy may be required. In the long term, the conventional criteria for managing ocular hypertension/glaucoma should be adopted, and surgical management will prove necessary for some patients (see chapter 9).

The cause of closed angle glaucoma needs to be defined, for example, a forward shift of the lens–iris diaphragm as may occur in posterior scleritis, or 360° posterior synechiae resulting from chronic anterior uveitis. The former may revert to normal with successful treatment of the scleritis whereas the latter requires laser peripheral iridotomy, and possibly trabeculectomy if IOP control cannot be obtained (see chapter 9).

Hypotony

Hypotony can result from a variety of different causes, the management of which is quite specific. Rhegmatogenous retinal detachment must be excluded, if necessary by ultrasonography if the fundal view is inadequate. Low pressure may result from excessive drainage in patients who have undergone filtration surgery for raised IOP/glaucoma. Three other major causes of hypotony also need to be considered: severe intraocular inflammation resulting in ciliary body failure, ciliary body detachment as a result of cyclitic membrane development, and the onset of phthisis. High resolution ultrasonography will identify ciliary body detachment, and a trial of maximum systemic therapy (that is, high dose steroids, together with a second line drug such as cyclosporin A) should then be considered to determine whether hypotension is reversible or not. In patients who do not respond to a trial of adequate immunosuppression, the drugs should be tapered to the lowest dose required to keep the inflammation under control and the eye comfortable. Ocular pain in a hypotonous eye can be a major management problem but enucleation is only rarely required. Topical steroid therapy is usually sufficient but retrobulbar alcohol injection may also prove helpful.

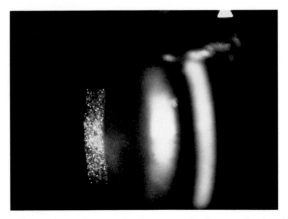

Figure 8.1   Posterior subcapsular lens opacity in a patients with uveitis.

Media opacities

Cataract is common in patients with uveitis, usually but not invariably posterior subcapsular in location (Fig 8.1) and often visually significant. In addition, other media opacities can occur, for example, posterior capsule opacification after cataract surgery with intraocular lens implantation, anterior pupillary membranes, and vitreous opacification secondary to vitritis, all of which can cause visual problems. Corneal oedema can result from endothelial dysfunction from a variety of causes: it may occur when keratic precipitates are extensively deposited over the endothelium, or as a result of drug induced endothelial decompensation, as has been observed with dorzolamide, the effects of which are reversible on withdrawal. Band keratopathy may be symptomatic from surface irregularity and visually disabling. Management of these complications frequently requires surgical intervention (see chapter 9).

Vitreous haemorrhage

There are many causes of vitreous haemorrhage in inflamed eyes whose management depends upon the underlying cause. If the fundus cannot be visualised as a result of dense haemorrhage, B scan ultrasonography is necessary to exclude retinal detachment. If the retina is flat, an expectant policy of observation can be followed, allowing the haemorrhage to clear and identifying the cause. Posterior vitreous detachment is the most common cause of vitreous haemorrhage in inflamed eyes, which may be associated

129

with retinal breaks, and lead to rhegmatogenous retinal detachment. This is, however, uncommon and in most situations the retina remains flat and the vitreous haemorrhage spontaneously resolves. Should this not occur, pars plana vitrectomy may be indicated. Retinal neovascularisation should always be suspected, and be carefully investigated for using fluorescein angiography if necessary. Posterior vitreous separation occurring in eyes with thickening of the posterior hyaloid face and increased vascular fragility as a result of uveitis are the most likely cause of vitreous haemorrhage when no specific aetiology can be identified.

Neovascularisation

In patients with posterior segment inflammation, neovascularisation can occur at a variety of sites and for several reasons. The two main causes are retinal ischaemia[42] and the severe inflammatory process itself.[43] It is very important to determine the aetiology of neovascularisation, by fluorescein angiography if necessary, so that appropriate therapy can be given. Patients may develop neovascularisation on the optic disc (NVD; Fig 8.2) or elsewhere in the retina (NVE) or in the subretinal space (SRN). Disorders that induce severe vasculitis with vascular closure, such as Eales' disease, and collagen diseases, such as Wegener's granulomatosis, tuberculosis, Behçet's disease, and sarcoidosis among others, may

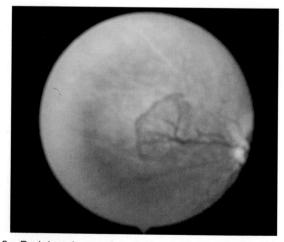

Figure 8.2 Peripheral vascular closure with "sea-fan" of new vessels arising from the optic disc.

result in areas of ischaemia as a result of either branch arterial or branch vein occlusion or peripheral vascular closure. Management of the neovascular response requires control of the inflammatory response but also ablative laser therapy to the ischaemic areas.

Subretinal neovascularisation can complicate any inflammatory process around chorioretinal lesions involving Bruch's membrane. Certain disorders such as presumed ocular histoplasmosis syndrome (POHS) (see chapter 7) are particularly associated with their formation,[45] in both the macular and peripapillary region, but they can occur in other disorders such as the Vogt–Koyanagi–Harada syndrome (see chapter 7) and toxoplasmosis (see chapter 5). Fluorescein angiography is mandatory to define the extent of the membrane and laser photocoagulation may be indicated, as in SRN occurring with age related macular degeneration. The inflammatory process should be controlled as well when active, but the membranes can occur at any time whether the inflammatory process is active or quiet (Fig 8.3). Consideration should be given to surgical removal of sub-foveal membranes in disorders such as POHS (see chapter 9).

Drug resistant macular oedema

Macular oedema remains the most common cause of irreversible visual loss in patients with uveitis (Fig 8.4). In many patients, it can be significantly ameliorated by immunosuppressive treatment, and bilateral macular oedema with severe visual impairment merits a trial of maximum therapy. Just occasionally, a patient is helped by oral carbonic anhydrase inhibitors and these are certainly worth a try.[46] Some patients with chronic macular oedema also develop epiretinal membranes which may merit surgical intervention. Two other forms of treatment are worth consideration, namely grid laser photocoagulation and pars plana vitrectomy (for vitrectomy, see chapter 9).

Macular-grid laser treatment has been shown to be beneficial in diabetic patients with non-ischaemic macular oedema and its use in macular oedema of chronic uveitis has been assessed in a recent study.[47] A temporary increase in oedema with paracentral scotomata was observed in the first few weeks but, after more than 18 months, macular oedema had been reduced significantly or disappeared as demonstrated by fluorescein angiography, in all the treated eyes. One eye had a significant increase in Snellen acuity, three eyes more or less stabilised, and two eyes deteriorated. The

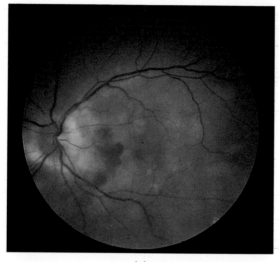

(a)

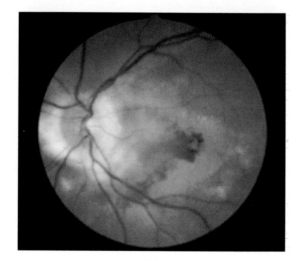

(b)

Figure 8.3 Peripapillary subretinal neovascular membrane in a quiet eye with old chorioretinal scars (a) showing progression when treated with increased immunosuppression alone (b).

role of such laser treatment in less intractable situations is unknown but the visual acuity results might be more favourable if performed at an earlier stage of the disease.

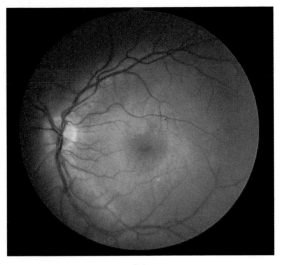

(a)

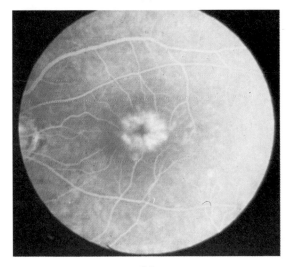

(b)

Figure 8.4 Macular oedema: (a) fundus photograph (b) fluorescein angiogram.

1 Rothova A, Suttorp-von Schulten MS, Frits Trefers WF, Kijlstra A. Causes and frequency of blindness in patients with intraocular inflammatory disease. *Br J Ophthalmol* 1996;**80**:332–6.
2 Lightman S. Use of steroids and immunosuppresive drugs in the management of uveitis. *Lancet* 1991;**338**:1501–4.

3 Lightman S, Chan C. Immune mechanisms in chorio-retinal inflammation in man. *Eye* 1990;4:345–53.

4 Riordan-Eva P, Lightman S. Orbital floor steroid injections in the treatment of posterior uveitis. *Eye* 1994;8:66–70.

5 Wakefield D, McCluskey P. Systemic immunosuppression in the treatment of posterior uveitis. *Int Ophthalmol Clin* 1995;35:107–22.

6 Wakefield D, McCluskey P, Penny R. Intravenous pulse methylprednisolone therapy in severe inflammatory eye disease. *Arch Ophthalmol* 1986;104:847–51.

7 de Smet MD, Nussenblatt RB. Clinical use of cyclosporine in ocular disease. *Int Ophthalmol Clin* 1993;33:31–45.

8 Whitcup SM, Salvo EC Jr, Nussenblatt RB. Combined cyclosporine and corticosteroid therapy for sight-threatening uveitis in Behçet's disease. *Am J Ophthalmol* 1994;118:39–45.

9 Vitale AT, Rodriguez A, Foster CS, de Smet MD. Low-dose cyclosporin A therapy in treating chronic, noninfectious uveitis *Ophthalmology* 1996;103:365–74.

10 Nussenblatt RB, Palestine AG, Chan CC, et al. Randomized, double-masked study of cyclosporine compared to prednisolone in the treatment of endogenous uveitis. *Am J Ophthalmol.* 1991;112:138–46.

11 De-Vries J, Baarsma GS, Zaal MJW, et al. Cyclosporin in the treatment of severe chronic idiopathic uveitis. *Br J Ophthalmol* 1990;74:344–9.

12 Towler HMA, Whiting PH, Forrester JV. Combination low dose Cyclosporin A and steroid therapy in chronic intraocular inflammation. *Eye* 1989;4:514-20.

13 Feutren G. Clinical experience with sandimmune (cyclosporine) in autoimmune diseases *Transplant Proc* 1992;24:55–60.

14 Hakin KN, Pearson RV, Lightman SL. Sympathetic ophthalmia: visual results with modern immunosuppressive therapy. *Eye* 1992;6:453–5.

15 Tabbara KF. Azathioprine in Behçet's syndrome (I). *N Engl J Med* 1990;323:195.

16 Rosenbaum JT. Treatment of severe refractory uveitis with intravenous cyclophosphamide. *J Rheumatol* 1994;21:123–5.

17 Palmer RG, Kanski JJ, Ansell BM. Chlorambucil in the treatment of intractable uveitis associated with juvenile chronic arthritis *J Rheumatol* 1985;12:967–70.

18 Tessler HH, Jennings T. High-dose short-term chlorambucil for intractable sympathetic ophthalmia and Behçet's disease. *Br J Ophthalmol* 1990;74:353–7.

19 Wilke WS, Biro JA, Segal AM. Methotrexate in the treatment of arthritis and connective tissue diseases. *Cleve Clin J Med* 1987;54:327–38.

20 Olsen NJ, Murray LM. Antiproliferative effects of methotrexate on peripheral blood monomuclear cells. *Arthritis Rheum* 1989;32:378–85.

21 Calabrese LH, Taylor JV, Wilke WS, et al. Response of immunoregulatory lymphocyte subsets to methotrexate in rheumatoid arthritis. *Cleve Clin J Med* 1990;57:232–41.

22 Holz FG, Krastel H, Breitbart A, Schwarz-Eywill M, Pezzutto A, Volcker HE. Low-dose methotrexate treatment in non-infectious uveitis resistant to corticosteroids. *German J Ophthalmol* 1992;1:142–4.

23 Shah SS, Lowder CY, Schmitt MA, Wilke WS, Kosmorsky GS, Meilser DM. Low-dose methotrexate therapy for ocular inflammatory disease. *Ophthalmology* 1992;99:1419–23.

24 Pascalis L, Pia G, Aresu G, Frongia T, Barca L. Combined cyclosporin A–steroid–MTX treatment in endogenous non-infectious uveitis. *J Autoimmun* 1993;6:467–80.

25 Mochizuki M, Masuda K, Sakane T, et al. A clinical trial of FK506 in refractory uveitis. *Am J Ophthalmol* 1993;115:763–9.

26 Sakane T, Mochizuki M, Inaba G, Masuda K. A phase II study of FK506 (tacrolimus) on refractory uveitis associated with Behçet's disease and allied conditions (Japanese). *Ryumachi* 1995;35:802–13.

27 Isioka M, Ohno S, Nakamura S, Isobe K, Watanabe N, Ishigatsubo Y, Tanaka S. FK506 treatment of non-infectious uveitis. *Am J Ophthalmol* 1994;**118**:723–9.
28 Hahn HJ. Kuttler B. Laube F. Emmrich F. Anti-CD4 therapy in recent-onset IDDM. *Diabetes Metab Rev* 1993;**9**:323–8.
29 Thurau SR, Wildner, G, Reiter C, Riethmuller G, Lund OE. Treatment of endogenous uveitis with anti-CD4 monoclonal antibody: first report. *German J Ophthalmol* 1994;**3**:409–13.
30 Nussenblatt RB, Caspi R, Mahdi C, Cahn C, Roberge F, Lider O, Weiner HL. Inhibition of S-antigen induced experimental autoimmune uveoretinitis by oral induction of tolerance with S-antigen. *J Immunol* 1990;**144**:1689–95.
31 Dick AD, Cheng YF, Liversidge J, Forrester JV. Intranasal administration of retinal antigens suppresses retinal antigen-induced experimental autoimmune uveoretinitis. *Immunology* 1994;**82**:625–31.
32 Nussenblatt RB, Whitcup SM, de Smet M, et al. Intraocular inflammatory disease (uveitis) and the use of oral tolerance: a status report. *Ann NY Acad Sci* 1996;**778**:325–37.
33 Hohol MJ, Khoury SJ, Cook S. et al. Three-year open protocol continuation study of oral tolerization with myelin antigens in multiple sclerosis and design of a phase III pivotal trial. *Ann NY Acad Sci* 1996;**778**:243–50.
34 Nussenblatt R, Gery I, Weiner H, et al. Treatment of uveitis by oral administration of retinal antigens: results of a phase 1/11 randomised masked trial. *Am J Ophthalmol* 1997;**123**:583–92.
35 Schulman JA, Peyman EA. Intravitreal corticosteroids as an adjunct in the treatment of bacterial and fungal endophthalmitis: a review. *Retina* 1992;**12**:336–340.
36 Stern GA. Factors affecting the efficacy of antibiotics in the treatment of experimental post-operative endophthalmitis. *Trans Am Ophthal* 1993;**91**:775–884.
37 Young SH, Morlet N, Heery St, et al. High dose intravitreal ganciclovir in the treatment of cytomegalovirus retinitis. *Med J Aust* 1992;**157**:370–3.
38 Anand R, Nightingale SD, Fish RH, et al. Control of cytomegalovirus retinitis using sustained release of intraocular ganciclovir. *Arch Ophthalmol* 1993;**111**:223.
39 Morley M, Duker J, Ashton P, Robinson M. Replacing ganciclovir implants. *Ophthalmology* 1995;**102**:388–92.
40 Cheng CK, Berger AS, Pearson PA, Ashton P, Jaffee GJ. Intravitreal sustained release dexamethasone device in the treatment of experimental uveitis. *Invest Ophthalmol Vis Sci* 1995;**36**:442–53.
41 Panek WC, Holland GN, Lee DA, Christensen R. Glaucoma in patients with uveitis. *Br J Ophthalmol* 1990;**74**:223–7.
42 Kwon YH, Dreyer EB. Inflammatory glaucomas. *Int Ophthalmol Clin* 1996;**36**:81–9.
43 Graham EM, Stanford MR, Schilling JS, Sanders DM. Neovascularisation associated with posterior uveitis. *Br J Ophthalmol* 1987;**71**:826–33.
44 Wakefield D, Lloyd A. The role of cytokines in the pathogenesis of inflammatory eye disease. *Cytokine* 1992;**4**:1–5.
45 Bottoni FG, Deutman AF, Aandekerk AL. Presumed ocular histoplasmosis syndrome and linear streak lesions. *Br J Ophthalmol* 1989;**73**:528–35.
46 Cox SN, Hay E, Bird AC. Treatment of chronic macular edema with acetazolamide. *Arch Ophthalmol* 1988;**106**:1190–5.
47 Suttorp-Schulten MS, Feron E, Postema F, Kijlstra A, Rothova A. Macular grid laser photocoagulation in uveitis. *Br J Ophthalmol* 1995;**79**:821–4.

9: Surgery in eyes with uveitis

Surgical intervention in eyes afflicted by uveitis can be considered within one of three broad categories: surgical treatment of a complication of uveitis or its therapy (for example, cataract), surgery as specific therapy for an inflammatory problem, (for example, macular oedema), and surgery to obtain tissue to establish a diagnosis (for example, by histopathology or microbial culture). In some circumstances, surgical procedures may be performed for several of these reasons.

PATIENT SELECTION AND PLANNING OF SURGERY

It is a generally accepted maxim that elective intraocular surgery in eyes with uveitis should be performed only when the inflammation is in complete remission.[1-3] In the ideal situation, there should be no signs of inflammatory activity and this is particularly appropriate for those patterns of uveitis characterised by well defined acute episodes, for example, acute anterior uveitis associated with HLA-B27. When the intraocular inflammation is of a more chronic and persistent pattern, such as the uveitis associated with juvenile chronic arthritis (JCA), complete abolition of intraocular inflammation may be achievable only through profound immunosuppression[4] which poses significant risks for the patient, and may not be absolutely necessary for a successful surgical outcome.[5, 6] The use of prophylactic corticosteroid therapy to suppress intraocular inflammation is widely endorsed, although the optimum regimen regarding dose, duration, and route of administration has not been universally defined (see below).

The absolute period of disease remission or suppression before elective surgery is a matter of debate among surgeons, but a minimum of three months of quiescence has broad acceptance. The timing of surgical intervention will also depend on individual patient factors, including the level of vision in the other eye, coexisting systemic inflammatory or other disorders, and social factors, for example, the educational needs of a child or young adult.

In those situations requiring diagnostic intervention, for example, suspected lymphoma or intraocular infection, it may be necessary to operate on an inflamed eye. The patient may already be receiving systemic steroids and shown a poor clinical response to treatment, raising the possibility of a masquerade syndrome.

PREOPERATIVE MANAGEMENT OF UVEITIS PATIENTS

The rationale of prophylactic anti-inflammatory therapy with systemic steroids is to reduce the risks of an inflammatory rebound in the posterior segment during the immediate postoperative period and optimise the outcome of surgery with minimum visual and systemic morbidity.

Eyes with inflammation confined to the anterior segment and with no history of macular oedema do not, as a rule, require prophylactic systemic steroids. When there has been a panuveitis or documented posterior segment involvement, steroid prophylaxis is indicated for cataract and posterior segment surgery. Glaucoma surgery appears to have a much lower risk of inflammatory rebound and prophylaxis is not usually required unless there has been an adverse inflammatory outcome after similar surgery in the fellow eye.

Steroid prophylaxis is not required in patients with Fuchs' heterochromic cyclitis[7] who require cataract surgery unless macular oedema has previously been confirmed, preferably by fluorescein angiography. Patients already receiving systemic steroids and/or immunosuppressive therapy such as cyclosporin A will usually need to increase their steroid dose before surgery because maintenance systemic treatment is normally kept to the minimum required to control inflammation.[3]

Prophylactic steroid therapy is started between one and two weeks before surgery at a dose of 0.5 mg/kg per day of pre-

UVEITIS

dnisolone[3] (or equivalent for other steroid preparations, for example, prednisone, methylprednisolone). This dose is maintained for about one week after surgery, then tapered according to clinical progress, with a reduction of 5 mg prednisolone per week usually being possible.

Intravenous steroid administration at the time of surgery has been used as an alternative to oral steroids, employing a dose of 500–1000 mg methylprednisolone. This is delivered by slow intravenous infusion, and can be repeated if necessary during the immediate postoperative period. The major risk from intravenous steroid infusion is acute cardiovascular collapse and caution should be exercised in older patients or if there is a history of cardiac disease.

Intravitreal steroid (dexamethasone) can be administered at the end of posterior segment surgery, but there are few published data on the value of this route of delivery in uveitis.[1, 8] The clearance of steroid from the vitreous cavity after vitrectomy is rapid and, although high levels can be achieved, these are very transient. A study of intravitreal injection of 800 μg dexamethasone after vitrectomy in eyes with proliferative diabetic retinopathy[8] showed a lower incidence of flare and fibrin in the anterior chamber in the treated group compared with controls. The introduction of slow release intravitreal steroid devices[9] may in future offer the prospect of intraocular surgery in uveitic eyes without systemic steroid prophylaxis or postoperative therapy.

POSTOPERATIVE MANAGEMENT

Anterior uveitis should be treated with topical steroids (for example, betamethasone, dexamethasone, or prednisolone acetate) given with sufficient frequency to control anterior chamber activity. The spectrum of activity will vary considerably between patients, typically being minimal in Fuchs' heterochromic cyclitis and greatest in eyes that have required the most iris manipulation. In uncomplicated procedures, four times daily administration will usually suffice, but after complex anterior segment surgery 1–2 hourly topical steroid drops should be used, then adjusted according to clinical progress. Topical non-steroidal anti-inflammatory agents (for example, indomethacin, ketorolac, flurbiprofen) can also be administered postoperatively.

138

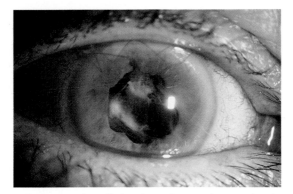

Figure 9.1 Postoperative fibrin deposits on intraocular lens implant surface after extracapsular cataract and pupil surgery.

Fibrin deposition in the anterior chamber, especially within the visual axis (Fig 9.1), is an indication for more intensive topical steroid therapy, and lysis with recombinant tissue plasminogen activator, for example, alteplase. This can be injected via a paracentesis and should be performed at an early stage before cellular invasion of the membrane occurs. Periocular depot steroid (triamcinolone or methylprednisolone) can also be administered unless the intraocular pressure is or has been elevated.

The presence of a hypopyon in the immediate postoperative period may be the result of severe inflammation or endophthalmitis. It is prudent to manage these eyes as suspected endophthalmitis, and to give intravitreal antibiotics (vancomycin 1–2 mg and amikacin 400 µg or ceftazidime 1 mg) after obtaining aqueous and vitreous samples.

SURGICAL TREATMENT OF THE COMPLICATIONS OF UVEITIS

Cataract

The development of cataract in eyes with uveitis is common and may occur as a result of both the inflammatory process and its treatment with topical, periocular, or systemic corticosteroids. Uveitis primarily affects young adults who have high visual requirements and, in the past, may have been advised against surgical intervention until the cataract was considerably advanced because of the significant risk of complications after intervention.

Although these risks have not been abolished, advances in surgical technique, better control of inflammation, careful patient selection, and meticulous perioperative management have significantly improved the outcome of surgery for uveitis related cataracts during the last 20 years.

Indications for cataract surgery

The most common indication for surgery is visual rehabilitation. In eyes with sufficient lens opacity to preclude an adequate view of the posterior segment, cataract surgery may prove necessary to allow monitoring of treatment of the underlying inflammation. Phacolytic glaucoma and lens induced uveitis are less common indications for lens extraction in eyes with established uveitis.

Surgical techniques

Phacoemulsification

Although there is a paucity of reliable data confirming that phacoemulsification has a lesser propensity to exacerbate inflammation in uveitic eyes, this is generally perceived to be the case, and is supported by studies in non-inflamed eyes.[10] Phacoemulsification has the advantage of a smaller entry wound and minimal or no conjunctival trauma, the second being particularly important if glaucoma filtration surgery has to be undertaken subsequently. In addition, there is now a wide variety of intraocular lens implants manufactured from different materials available which may have specific advantages in eyes with uveitis (see below). Except in the most severely bound down pupil, it is usually possible to enlarge the pupil sufficiently to perform an adequate capsulorrhexis which is the most critical element during this type of surgery in uveitic eyes. Fibrosis of the anterior capsule with subsequent constriction (capsular phimosis or capsular contraction syndrome[11]) occurs more commonly in eyes with uveitis, and the risk of this developing can be avoided by performing a generous capsulorrhexis either at the time of the primary capsulorrhexis or by enlarging the capsulorrhexis after implantation of a lens.

Extracapsular and intercapsular

Extracapsular cataract extraction remains an important surgical method, particularly where phacoemulsification facilities are less readily available and uveitis is common, for example, in the developing world. Although the extracapsular approach offers good access to the pupil, refinements in the surgical techniques for managing small pupils during phacoemulsification have reduced the need to use the extracapsular approach solely for this reason. The larger wound is more prone to cause problems during combined procedures, for example, fluid leak when combined with pars plana vitrectomy, and the slower rate of visual recovery[3] compared with phacoemulsification is frustrating for patients.

Lensectomy

Lensectomy is most frequently performed when cataract surgery is combined with pars plana vitrectomy. It remains the method of choice for removal of cataracts in JCA related uveitis when an anterior or complete vitrectomy is also performed to prevent the development of a cyclitic membrane and subsequent hypotony.[5, 6] In JCA related uveitis eyes with cataract and mobile pupils, phacoemulsification can be undertaken accompanied by intra-ocular lens implantation. Lensectomy has been almost superseded by phacoemulsification when combined vitrectomy and cataract surgery is undertaken in other patterns of uveitis because good capsular support for an intraocular lens is retained and a deep anterior chamber can easily be maintained during the vitrectomy, thus facilitating insertion of a lens implant at the end of the procedure if indicated.[12] Lensectomy does allow retention of the anterior capsule to support a lens implant, either as a primary or secondary procedure.

Management of small pupils

Careful management of the small pupil is the key to success in uveitis cataract and vitreoretinal surgery. Stripping of fibrous bands around the pupil margin may allow sufficient enlargement of the pupil to give reasonable access to the lens. If this is insufficient and stretching of the iris sphincter does not result in an adequate pupillary aperture, multiple small sphincterotomies (Fig 9.2) can be performed with capsule scissors or retinal scissors; the retinal scissors have the advantage of allowing access through the side port incision during phacoemulsification. It is important to avoid large iridotomies if phacoemulsification is planned because this will result in mobile tags of iris which are easily aspirated into and traumatised by the tip of the phacoemulsification probe. Where extracapsular or intercapsular lens extraction is planned, the iridotomies can be more generous, and a large, superior radial iridotomy will also allow excellent access to the lens; this iridotomy can subsequently be sutured with polypropylene to improve cosmesis and reduce the problems associated with a large and

141

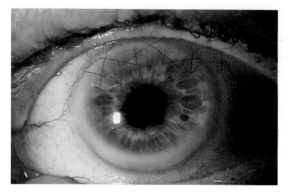

Figure 9.2 Extracapsular cataract surgery with multiple small inferior sphincterotomies.

irregular pupil (Fig 9.3).

Self retaining iris retractors have become popular for maintaining an adequate pupil during cataract and vitreoretinal surgery. It is important not to stretch the pupil excessively with the retractors because radial tears of the iris may occur (Fig 9.4), especially if fibrosis involves only a sector of the pupil. Iris retractors are particularly useful when combined cataract extraction and vitrectomy is planned, although the retractors can be easily dislocated if an irrigating contact lens is used. During lensectomy, the vitreous cutter can also be used to enlarge the pupil if iris retractors are not available, although care should be taken to avoid removing excessive iris tissue.

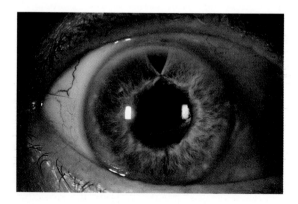

Figure 9.3 Endocapsular cataract surgery with sutured superior radial iridotomy and inferior sphincterotomies.

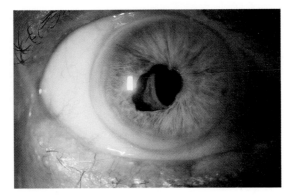

Figure 9.4 Inferotemporal iris tear after the use of self retaining iris hooks for phacoemulsification in chronic anterior uveitis.

It is important to minimise trauma to the iris as much as possible, because bleeding from the iris will lead to the deposition of fibrin at the pupil and on the lens implant if present. This increases the risk of synechiae formation to the edge of the anterior capsule and pupillary membrane development. Postoperative fibrin deposition in the anterior chamber is best treated by the injection of recombinant tissue plasminogen activator (rtPA, 5–25 μg in 100 μl), in combination with mydriatics and intensive topical steroids. Injections of rtPA can be repeated if fibrin deposition recurs.

Lens materials

Although there have been exciting developments in intraocular lens technology, the ideal material for lens implants in eyes with uveitis has not yet been identified. Small cellular deposits and giant cells can be observed on the intraocular lens implant surface in normal eyes after cataract surgery[13] and these changes are more marked in uveitic eyes.[14] Heparin surface modification of polymethyl methacrylate (PMMA) lenses reduces the number and extent of these deposits but does not completely prevent their formation.[7] Acrylic and hydrogel lens implants are associated with fewer surface deposits than unmodified PMMA lenses and these materials are flexible, which allows the lens to be foldable. Although silicone lenses are foldable, their tendency to develop surface deposits lies somewhere between PMMA and acrylic or hydrogel implants. The surface of all types of lens implants can be damaged by rough or injudicious handling during insertion which may neutralise the benefits of any particular lens type.[15]

143

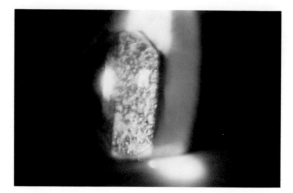

Figure 9.5   Extensive cellular deposits on a PMMA intraocular lens implant.

Lens deposits are more likely to occur in eyes where there is continuing inflammatory activity, for example, in chronic anterior uveitis or Fuchs' heterochromic cyclitis (Fig 9.5). The deposits can be "polished" off the lens surface by low energy neodymium: yttrium–aluminium–garnet (Nd:YAG) laser, although care must be exercised to avoid pitting the surface which may promote further cellular deposition.

Posterior capsule opacification (PCO)

This is more common in uveitic eyes primarily because of the younger age of patients[16, 17] and this tendency may be exacerbated by some lens materials and designs. Acrylic lenses appear to have the lowest propensity to cause posterior capsule opacification (PCO), in comparison to PMMA and hydrogel lenses. Posterior capsule opacification is related not only to the material from which the lens is manufactured, but also to the design of the lens and the degree of contact between the optic and the posterior capsule.[16]

Posterior capsule opacification can usually be treated by Nd:YAG laser capsulotomy as for non-uveitic eyes. Laser capsulotomy should not be undertaken when there is active intraocular inflammation because there is a risk of inducing or exacerbating macular oedema. Post-laser intraocular pressure rise should be minimised by treatment with apraclonidine drops. A significant number of uveitic eyes with PCO also have opacification of the anterior vitreous face, which may be adherent to the posterior capsule and laser capsulotomy may fail to divide this adequately. In this situation, posterior capsulectomy and anterior vitrectomy may be required via a pars plana approach.

An increase in uveitis after Nd:YAG laser capsulotomy may reflect increased endogenous inflammatory activity, but, especially in the presence of hypopyon, low grade, delayed, postoperative endophthalmitis caused by organisms such as *Propionibacterium acnes* or *Staphylococcus epidermidis* must be borne in mind, and appropriate intraocular tissue samples obtained for culture (see later).

There is no conclusive evidence that the type of material used for the intraocular lens implant has any influence on the development of macular oedema. A recent comparative study[18] of acrylic and silicone lens implants, in combined cataract and glaucoma surgery in non-uveitic eyes, demonstrated higher intraocular pressure, particularly in the immediate postoperative period in the acrylic lens group. It is important, therefore, that the surgeon remains vigilant for potential problems when using newer lens materials in "at-risk" eyes.

Glaucoma

Raised intraocular pressure is common in eyes with uveitis and may affect up to 20% or more of such patients.[19] Sustained elevation of intraocular pressure leading to secondary glaucoma most frequently occurs in association with chronic inflammation involving the anterior segment, which may occur in isolation or as part of a panuveitis.[20] Acute anterior uveitis may also be associated with raised intraocular pressure, but this is more often self limiting and resolves with control of the uveitis.[21] The management of raised intraocular pressure and glaucoma in uveitis presents a number of difficulties. Many of these eyes have chronic ongoing inflammation, and cessation of topical steroids may not be possible, even where there is a clearly defined steroid responsive element to the elevated intraocular pressure. In addition to uveitis, there may be additional risk factors for treatment failure such as aphakia or pseudophakia,[22] black ethnic origin,[23] young age,[24] and prolonged duration of antiglaucoma therapy.[25]

Topical hypotensive therapy in uveitis related glaucoma has, until recently, been largely restricted to the use of β blockers, and when these have proved inadequate, systemic therapy with

145

carbonic anhydrase inhibitors (CAI), such as acetazolamide or dichlorphenamide, was usually introduced. Miotics and adrenergic agents are of limited value in uveitis related glaucoma, although they may be helpful in the short term in controlling intraocular pressure. The recent introduction of prostaglandin agonists such as latanoprost,[26] the α_2 agonists apraclonidine and brimonidine, and the topical CAI dorzolamide may offer alternative topical drug regimens to improve control of intraocular pressure, but specific clinical studies of these new agents in uveitis related glaucoma have not been undertaken. When medical therapy fails to control intraocular pressure satisfactorily, surgery is usually required. Unfortunately, the success rate of conventional filtration surgery, such as trabeculectomy, has been reported to range from 58% to 75%, and alternative surgical procedures such as trabeculodialysis have been recommended.[26, 27] During the last five years, filtration surgery with an antimetabolite (5-fluorouracil [5FU][28–31] or mitomycin C [MMC][32, 33]) has become an increasingly popular method of controlling uveitis related glaucoma, although the need for these agents has been disputed.[34, 35] Some of the reported differences in outcome after filtration surgery reflect selection bias, small sample sizes, and population differences. Aphakia, pseudophakia, and black ethnic origin do appear to carry a significantly increased risk of failure of conventional filtration surgery, and these patients should be offered antimetabolite therapy with filtration surgery. Therapy with MMC may offer slightly better pressure control than 5FU, but is associated with a higher incidence of postoperative hypotony[36] and the long term risks of leaking and avascular blebs has not yet been reliably determined in these relatively young eyes.

Seton drains, for example the Molteno drain,[37] are a useful surgical option in very high risk eyes, particularly aphakic eyes (Fig 9.6) and in JCA associated uveitis with secondary glaucoma. The drain can be implanted as a one or two stage procedure, and can be undertaken as a primary procedure or when conventional filtration surgery has failed.

Transscleral Nd:YAG or diode laser cyclophotocoagulation has, to some extent, superseded transscleral cyclocryopexy for pressure control in intractable glaucoma from other causes such as neovascularisation.[38, 39] There are no comparative studies of laser cyclophotocoagulation with seton drainage in uveitis, but a recent comparative study in neovascular glaucoma demonstrated greater success with surgery.[40]

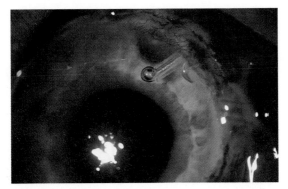

Figure 9.6   Molteno drain in aphakic eye with chronic anterior uveitis and failed trabeculectomy. Note the small gas bubble (C_3F_8) used to prevent hypotony in the immediate postoperative period.

Vitreoretinal complications

Vitreous opacification

Although vitreous hase is common in eyes with uveitis, it is not a major cause of serious visual problems for most patients unless there is coexisting, visually significant cataract or macular oedema. Quite striking and symptomatic vitreous changes may develop in Fuchs' heterochromic cyclitis, and these can be cleared by pars plana vitrectomy, often in combination with cataract surgery.

Epiretinal membranes

The management of epiretinal membranes (ERMs) follows similar principles to those in non-inflamed eyes (Fig 9.7). It may be difficult clinically to discriminate between macular oedema and mild retinal surface wrinkling (cellophane maculopathy), and fluorescein angiography should be undertaken to establish this. Angiography will also help to confirm the need for steroid prophylaxis which, in general, will usually be needed for any posterior segment surgery. Toxoplasma chorioretinitis in particular is associated with very severe postoperative inflammation, and it is important not to reduce steroid therapy too quickly after surgery.

Egpiretinal membranes may, on occasion, undergo spontaneous resolution in uveitic eyes as a result of posterior vitreous separation, in contrast to idiopathic age related ERM where the posterior vitreous has usually already detached. For this reason, ERM associated with an attached vitreous may be observed until

147

posterior vitreous detachment occurs, unless surgical removal is indicated for visual reasons.

Vitreous haemorrhage and retinal neovascularisation

Retinal neovascularisation can develop in uveitis either as a direct result of the inflammatory process or secondary to retinal

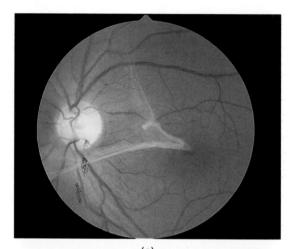

(a)

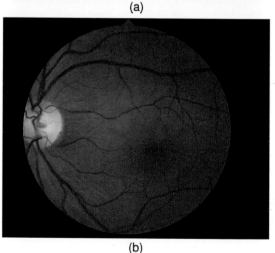

(b)

Figure 9.7 (a) Epiretinal membrane attached to fovea in eye with toxoplasma chorioretinitis. (b) Postoperative appearance after vitrectomy and membrane peel. Visual acuity improved from 6/18 to 6/6.

ischaemia, for example, in Eales' disease. Neovascularisation may lead to vitreous haemorrhage which tends to be self limiting but may require pars plana vitrectomy with endolaser photocoagulation if it fails to clear spontaneously. Fluorescein angiography is usually necessary to determine the pathogenesis of neovascularisation in order to allow appropriate therapy because inflammatory neovascularisation should be treated by immunosuppression in the first instance, in contrast to neovascularisation secondary to retinal ischaemia which requires laser photocoagulation similar to proliferative diabetic retinopathy.

Subretinal neovascularisation

Subretinal neovascular membranes may develop in any pattern of uveitis that results in chorioretinal scarring, and subfoveal neovascularisation is a particular feature of the presumed ocular histoplasmosis syndrome (POHS) and punctate inner choroidopathy (Fig 9.8). Other patterns of uveitis more commonly associated with subretinal neovascularisation include sympathetic ophthalmia, birdshot choroidoretinopathy, and toxoplasma chorioretinitis. In POHS, 76% of eyes with subfoveal neovascular membranes have a visual acuity of 6/60 or less within two years, with only 12% showing spontaneous recovery of 2 Snellen lines.[41, 42]

Subfoveal membranes may be surgically removed with reasonable prospects of visual improvement, especially in POHS in contrast to the results of intervention in age related macular degeneration. This is thought to occur because the retinal pigment epithelium (RPE) is less likely to be removed with inflammatory membranes as the neovascular complex is situated between the neurosensory retina and the RPE. About one in three eyes with POHS and subfoveal neovascularisation obtained visual improvement of 2 Snellen lines or more, with 44% experiencing no significant change in acuity (±1 Snellen line).[43] The visual results of surgical excision were poorer in older patients and if the membranes had previously been treated by laser photocoagulation. Recurrence of membranes after surgery remains a problem affecting 38% of eyes in this series, and is associated with a poor visual prognosis. Subretinal neovascularisation does not usually respond to immunosuppressive therapy, and other therapeutic options (for example, radiotherapy, intravitreal steroid injection) are still being assessed.

Tractional and rhegmatogenous retinal detachment

Chronic intraocular inflammation involving the posterior segment causes vitreous changes that, through their tractional effects on the retina, may lead to tractional retinal detachment, retinal tears, and ultimately rhegmatogenous retinal detachment. These detachments may be amenable to repair by conventional retinal surgery but pars plana vitrectomy allows clearance of media opacity with relief of vitreous traction. Rhegmatogenous retinal detachment has been associated with transscleral cryopexy per-

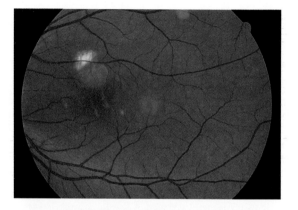

(a)

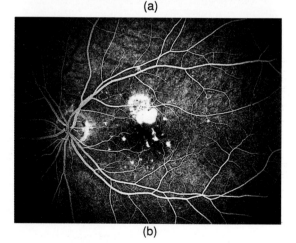

(b)

Figure 9.8 (a) Presumed ocular histoplasmosis syndrome with juxtafoveal choroidal neovascular membrane, adjacent to pale atrophic area; (b) Late venous phase fluorescein angiogram.

formed for peripheral retinal and snowbank neovascularisation in pars planitis.

SURGERY AS SPECIFIC THERAPY FOR INFLAMMATORY COMPLICATIONS

Therapeutic vitrectomy

It has become evident during the last 20 years that some eyes will show a dramatic clinical and visual response to vitrectomy even when immunosuppressive medical therapy has been unrewarding.[1, 44-51] Pars planitis and intermediate uveitis in particular may respond well to surgical treatment but this response does not appear to be related to either the duration of disease or the preoperative visual acuity. The mechanisms by which vitrectomy leads to improvement in macular oedema are unknown but are thought to be related to increased clearance of inflammatory mediators and leucocytes from the vitreous cavity after vitrectomy.

Neovascularisation of the peripheral snowbanks

This occurs in pars planitis and can be treated by transscleral cryopexy, or pars plana vitrectomy combined with peripheral endolaser photocoagulation or cryopexy. Although cryopexy is popular in North America for second line treatment of pars planitis, it has never achieved the same popularity in the United Kingdom, where systemic steroids are often used in preference. Although there is a considerable amount of anecdotal support for a role for vitrectomy in uveitis, there are no randomised controlled trials of vitrectomy versus medical therapy in pars planitis or other patterns of inflammation.

Band keratopathy

This is a frequent finding in eyes with long standing chronic inflammation (Fig 9.9), for example, in JCA associated uveitis. If symptomatic because of either impaired visual acuity or surface irregularity and discomfort, it can be removed by chelation with ethylenediamine tetraacetic acid (EDTA) or ablated by superficial phototherapeutic keratectomy (PTK) with excimer laser.

151

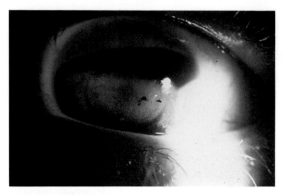

Figure 9.9   Band keratopathy in a child with uveitis associated with juvenile chronic arthritis.

DIAGNOSTIC PROCEDURES

Biopsy of intraocular tissues of eyes with uveitis may be valuable in establishing an infective or neoplastic aetiology, or in confirming a specific inflammatory cause. Antibodies in fluids can be quantitatively measured, for examples by enzyme linked immuno-sorbent assay (ELISA), and cells may analysed by immunocytochemistry, cytopathology, flow cytometry[52] by fluorescence activated cell sorter (FACS) analysis, and conventional staining. Selective biopsies of iris, retina, or choroid may be obtained for histopathology and immunocytochemistry, particularly when considering a diagnosis of intraocular lymphoma. Bacteriological assessment of intraocular fluids by culture and polymerase chain reaction (PCR)[53] may be conclusive when underlying infection is considered, for example, delayed post-operative endophthalmitis caused by organisms of low virulence such as *P acnes* and *Staph epidermidis*.

Aqueous biopsy

Antibody levels in the aqueous can be measured in a paracentesis sample and compared with serum antibody levels. These are then expressed in relation to albumin and total immunoglobulin concentrations (modified Witmer coefficient) which may indicate local, that is intraocular, antibody synthesis. This may be valuable in toxoplasmosis, toxocariasis, and herpes virus associated patterns of uveitis.[54]

Vitreous biopsy

Cellular analysis, microbiological culture, PCR analysis, and cytokine (especially interleukin 10, II-10) measurement of vitreous samples may be extremely helpful in distinguishing infectious and neoplastic vitreous infiltration from endogenous inflammation. Samples of 250–500 μl may be obtained by a needle biopsy via the pars plana, but larger vitreous biopsies should be undertaken by pars plana vitrectomy when 1–2 ml, of undiluted vitreous can readily be collected. A single use, 23 G disposable, vitreous cutter is also available for vitreous sampling.

Iris biopsy

It is uncommon to need to biopsy the iris in uncomplicated uveitis but when there are unusual clinical features or malignancy is suspected, iris biopsy can prove definitive.

Chorioretinal biopsy

This can be undertaken by the transscleral or endoretinal routes. The transscleral approach provides good access for peripheral lesions and allows a more generous size of specimen, but may be inaccurate if the target lesion is small. Endoretinal biopsy allows much more accurate localisation of pathology but provides very small tissue samples which may be difficult to process and interpret with conventional histopathological techniques, although recent developments in PCR and immunocytochemistry have considerably enhanced the value of this approach.

1 Diamond JG, Kaplan HJ. Lensectomy and vitrectomy for complicated cataract secondary to uveitis. *Arch Ophthalmol* 1978;**96**:1798–804.
2 Foster CS, Fong LP, Singh G. Cataract surgery and intraocular lens implantation in patients with uveitis. *Ophthalmology* 1989;**96**:281–8.
3 Barton K, Hall AJH, Rosen PH, Cooling RJ, Lightman S. Systemic steroid prophylaxis for cataract surgery in patients with uveitis. *Ocular Immunol Inflamm* 1994;**2**:207–216.
4 Ceisler EJ, Foster CS. Juvenile rheumatoid arthritis and uveitis: Minimizing the blinding complications. *Int Ophthalmol Clin* 1996;**36**:91–107.
5 Kanski JJ. Lensectomy for complicated cataract in juvenile chronic iridocyclitis. *Br J Ophthalmol* 1992;**76**:72–5.
6 Flynn HW Jr, Davis JL, Culbertson WW. Pars plana lensectomy and vitrectomy for complicated cataracts in juvenile rheumatoid arthritis. *Ophthalmology* 1988;**95**:1114–19.

7 Jones NP. Cataract surgery using heparin surface-modified intraocular lenses in Fuchs' heterochromic uveitis. *Ophthal Surg* 1995;**26**:49–52.

8 Blankenship GW. Evaluation of a single intravitreal injection of dexamethasone phosphate in vitrectomy surgery for diabetic retinopathy complications. *Graefe's Arch Clin Exp Ophthalmol* 1991;**229**:62–5.

9 Cheng CK, Berger AS, Pearson PA, Ashton P, Jaffe GJ. Intravitreal sustained-release dexamethasone device in the treatment of experimental uveitis. *Invest Ophthalmol Vis Sci* 1995;**36**:442–53.

10 Oshika T, Yoshimura K, Miyata N. Postsurgical inflammation after phacoemulsification and extracapsular extraction with soft or conventional intraocular lens implantation. *J Cataract Refract Surg* 1992;**18**:356–61.

11 Davison JA. Capsule contraction syndrome. *J Cataract Refracts Surg* 1993;**19**:582–9.

12 Koenig SB, Mieler WF, Han DP, Abrams GW. Combined phacoemulsification, pars plana vitrectomy, and posterior chamber intraocular lens insertion. *Arch Ophthalmol* 1992;**110**:1101–4.

13 Shah SM, Spalton DJ. Comparison of the postoperative inflammatory response in the normal eye with heparin-surface-modified and poly(methyl methacrylate) intraocular lenses. *J Cataract Refracts Surg* 1995;**21**:579–85.

14 Percival SPB, Pai V. Heparin-modified lenses for eyes at risk for breakdown of the blood aqueous barrier during cataract surgery. *J Cataract Refracts Surg* 1993;**19**:760–5.

15 Dick B, Kohnen T, Jacobi KW. Alterationen der Heparinbeschichtung auf Intraokularlinsen durch Implantationsinstrumente. *Klin Monatsbl Augenheilkd* 1995;**206**:460–6.

16 Apple DJ, Solomon KD, Tetz MR, et al. Posterior capsule opacification. *Surv Ophthalmol* 1992;**37**:73–116.

17 Dana MR, Chatzistefanou K, Schaumberg DA, Foster CS. Posterior capsule opacification after cataract surgery in patients with uveitis. *Ophthalmology* 1997;**104**:1387–94.

18 Lemon LC, Shin DH, Man SS, Lee JH, Bendel RE, Juzych MS, Hughes BA. Comparative study of silicone versus acrylic foldable lens implantation in primary glaucoma triple procedure. *Ophthalmology* 1997;**104**:178–13.

19 Panek WC, Holland GN, Lee DA, Christensen RE. Glaucoma in patients with uveitis. *Br J Ophthalmol* 1990;**74**:223–7.

20 Ritch R. Pathophysiology of glaucoma in uveitis. *Trans Ophthalmol Soc UK* 1981;**100**:321–4.

21 Krupin T, Feitl ME. Glaucoma associated with uveitis. In: Ritch R, Shields MB, Krupin T. *The Glaucomas*, Vol 2. St. Louis: CV Mosby, 1989:1209.

22 Heuer DK, Gressel MG, Parrish RK II, Anderson DR, Hodapp E, Palmberg PF. Trabeculectomy in aphakic eyes. *Ophthalmology* 1984;**94**:1045–51.

23 Wilson R, Richardson TM, Hertzmark E, Grant WM. Race as a risk factor for progressive glaucomatous damage. *Ann Ophthalmol* 1985;**17**:653–9.

24 Stürmer J, Broadway DC, Hitchings RA. Young patient trabeculectomy. Assessment of risk factors for failure. *Ophthalmology* 1993;**100**:928–39.

25 Lavin MJ, Wormald RPL, Migdal CS, Hitchings RA. The influence of prior therapy on the success of trabeculectomy. *Arch Ophthalmol* 1990;**108**:1543–8.

26 Mishima H, Kitazawa Y, Masuda K. Ocular hypotensive effect of PhXA41 in patients with ocular hypertension or primary open-angle glaucoma. *Jpn J Ophthalmol.* 1993;**37**:270–4.

27 Hoskins HD, Hetherington J, Shjaffer RN. Surgical management of the inflammatory glaucomas. *Perspect Ophthalmol* 1977;**1**:173–81.

28 Kanski JJ, Shun–Shin GA. Systemic uveitis syndromes in childhood : an analysis of 340 cases. *Ophthalmology* 1984;**91**:1247–51.

29 Jampel HD, Jabs DA, Quigley HA. Trabeculectomy with 5-fluorouracil for adult inflammatory glaucoma. *Am J Ophthalmol* 1990;**109**:168–73.

30 Ruderman SM, Welch DB, Smith MF, Schoch DE. A randomised study of 5-Fluorouracil and filtration surgery. *Am J Ophthalmol,* 1987;**104**:218–24.

31 The Fluorouracil Filtering Surgery Study Group. Fluorouracil filtering surgery study one-year follow-up. *Am J Ophthalmol.* 1989;**108**:625–35.

32 Chen CW, Huang HT, Bair JS, Lee CC. Trabeculectomy with simultaneous topical application of mitomycin-C in refractory glaucoma. *J Ocul Pharmacol* 1990;**6**:175–82.

33 Skuta GL, Beeson CC, Higginbotham EJ et al. Intraoperative mitomycin versus postoperative 5-fluorouracil in high-risk glaucoma filtering surgery. *Ophthalmology* 1992;**99**:438–44.

34 Towler HMA, Bates AK, Broadway DC, Lightman S. Primary trabeculectomy with 5-fluorouracil for glaucoma secondary to uveitis. *Ocul Immunol Inflamm* 1995;**3**:163–70.

35 Stavrou P, Misson GP, Rowson NJ, Murray PI. Trabeculectomy in uveitis. Are antimetabolites necessary as a first procedure? Ocul Immunol Inflamm 1995;**3**:209–16.

36 Shields MB, Scroggs, MW, Sloop, CM, Simmons RB. Clinical and histopatho-logical observations concerning hypotony after trabeculectomy with adjunctive mitomycin C. *Am J Ophthalmol* 1993;**116**:673–83.

37 Hill RA, Nguyen QH, Baerveldt G, et al. Trabeculectomy and Molteno Implantation for glaucomas associated with uveitis. Ophthalmology 1993;**100**:903–8.

38 Bloom PA, Tsai JC, Sharma K, Miller MH, Rice NSC, Hitchings RA, Khaw PT. "Cyclodiode": trans-scleral diode laser cyclophotocoagulation in the treatment of advanced refractory glaucoma. *Ophthalmology* 1997;**104**:1508–18.

39 Shields MB, Shields SE, Kass MA, Stark W, Taylor H. Noncontact transscleral ND:YAG cyclophotocoagulation: A long-term follow-up of 500 patients. *Trans Am Ophthalmol Soc* 1994;**92**:271–87.

40 Eid TE, Katz LJ, Spaeth GL, Augsburger JJ. Tube-shunt surgery versus Neodymium:YAG cyclophotocoagulation in the management of neovascular glaucoma. *Ophthalmology* 1997;**104**:1692–700.

41 Olk RJ, Burgess DB, McCormick PA. Subfoveal and juxtafoveal subretinal neovascularisation in the presumed ocular histoplasmosis syndrome. *Ophthal-mology* 1984;**91**:1592–602.

42 Fine SL, Wood WJ, Singerman LJ, et al. Laser treatment for subretinal neovascular membranes in ocular histoplasmosis syndrome: results of a pilot randomized clinical trial. *Arch Ophthalmol* 1993;**111**:19–20.

43 Berger AS, Conway M, Del Priore LV, Walker RS, Pollack JS, Kaplan HJ. Submacular surgery for subfoveal choroidal neovascular membranes in patients with presumed ocular histoplasmosis. *Arch Ophthalmol* 1997;**115**:991–996.

44 Diamond JG, and Kaplan HJ. Uveitis: effect of vitrectomy combined with lensectomy, *Ophthalmology* 1979;**86**:1320–7.

45 Limon S, deKyvon Y, Furia M, and Bloch–Michel E. La vitrectomie au cours des uvéites. Indications et résultats. *Bull Mem Soc Fr Ophthalmol* 1982;**94**:290–3.

46 Mieler WF, Will BR, Lewis H, Aaberg TM. Vitrectomy in the management of peripheral uveitis. *Ophthalmology* 1988;**95**:859–64.

47 Kloti R. Pars-plana Vitrektomie bei chronischer Uveitis. *Klin Monatsbl Augen-heilkd* 1988;**192**:425–9.

48 Berg P, Kroll P, Busse H. Surgical treatment of uveitis. *Klin Monatsbl Augenheilkd* 1990;**197**:373–7.

49 Bovey EH, Gonvers M, Herbort CP. Vitrectomie par la pars plana au cours des uveites. *Klin Monatsbl Augenheilkd* 1992;**200**:464–7.

50 Heiligenhaus A, Bornfeld N, Foerster MH, Wessing A. Long term results of pars plana vitrectomy in the management of complicated uveitis. *Br J Ophthalmol* 1994;**78**:549–54.

51 Verbraeken H. Therapeutic pars plana vitrectomy for chronic uveitis: A retrospective study of the long-term results. *Graefe's Arch Clin Exp Ophthalmol* 1996;**234**:288–93.

52 Freeman WR, Char DH, Garovoy MR, Lyon H. Microtechniques for flow cytometric analysis of aqueous humor lymphocytes. *J Immunol Methods* 1984;**73**:447–55.

53 Hykin PG, Tobal K, McIntyre G, Matheson MM, Towler H, Lightman S. The diagnosis of delayed post-operative endophthalmitis by polymerase chain reaction of bacterial DNA in vitreous samples. *J Med Microbiol* 1994;**44**:408–15.

54 Pepose JS, Flowers B, Stewart JA, Grose C, Levy DS, Culbertson WW, Kreiger AE. Herpesvirus antibody levels in the etiologic diagnosis of the acute retinal necrosis syndrome. *Am J Ophthalmol* 1992;**113**:248–56.

Index